Talking Therapy

Critical Issues in Health and Medicine

Edited by Rima D. Apple, University of Wisconsin–Madison and Janet Golden, Rutgers University–Camden

Growing criticism of the U.S. healthcare system is coming from consumers, politicians, the media, activists, and healthcare professionals. Critical Issues in Health and Medicine is a collection of books that explores these contemporary dilemmas from a variety of perspectives, among them political, legal, historical, sociological, and comparative, and with attention to crucial dimensions such as race, gender, ethnicity, sexuality, and culture.

For a list of titles in the series, see the last page of the book.

Talking Therapy

Knowledge and Power in American Psychiatric Nursing

Kylie M. Smith

Rutgers University Press

New Brunswick, Camden, and Newark, New Jersey, and London

Library of Congress Cataloging-in-Publication Data

Names: Smith, Kylie M., author.
Title: Talking therapy : knowledge and power in American psychiatric nursing /
    Kylie M. Smith.
Description: New Brunswick : Rutgers University Press, 2020. | Series: Critical issues
    in health and medicine | Includes bibliographical references and index.
Identifiers: LCCN 2019033148 (print) | LCCN 2019033149 (ebook) |
    ISBN 9781978801455 (paperback) | ISBN 9781978801462 (hardback) |
    ISBN 9781978801479 (epub)
Subjects: MESH: Psychiatric Nursing—history | Nurse's Role—history | Nurse-Patient
    Relations | History, 20th Century | United States Classification: LCC RC440 (print) |
    LCC RC440 (ebook) | NLM WY 11 AA1 | DDC 616.89/0231—dc23
LC record available at https://lccn.loc.gov/2019033148
LC ebook record available at https://lccn.loc.gov/2019033149

A British Cataloging-in-Publication record for this book is available from the British Library.

⊖ The paper used in this publication meets the requirements of the American National
Standard for Information Sciences—Permanence of Paper for Printed Library Materials,
ANSI Z39.48-1992.

www.rutgersuniversitypress.org

Manufactured in the United States of America

For Leah and Rachel Friedman, who survived.

Contents

Talking Therapy

Where Are the Nurses in the History of Psychiatry?

Before there were psychiatrists, there were "alienists." In 1894 Dr. Edward Cowles, the medical superintendent of the McLean Hospital for the Insane in Waverly, Massachusetts, delivered a paper to the meeting of the American Medico-Psychological Association celebrating its first twenty-five years. In his presentation, he referred repeatedly to "we American alienists," charting the progress of those physicians concerned with the mental and nervous diseases, who, starting with Founding Father Dr. Benjamin Rush, had sought to eliminate diseases of the mind through "blisters, issues, salivation, emetics, purges and a reduced diet."[1] If insanity had not been cured through exorcisms, chains, and restraints, Rush theorized that it may instead be eliminated through the blood or bodily fluids. He was of course largely wrong, and his successors in the 1890s knew that, but they were no closer to a cure than he had been. Alienists practiced their craft through trial and error, but always on the principle that the patient must be removed from their family, from the community, and from stressful environments. Alienated, if you will. Of course, this is not the dictionary meaning of "alienist"; etymologically it comes from the French *aliéniste*, referring to a doctor who treats the insane, which in turn was derived from the Latin *alius*, meaning "other"[2]—which can be interpreted as a reference to both the "other" of the insane, the "not normal," and the duality of those living with delusions, the "seeing of others." American alienists largely stopped calling themselves that when they changed the name of their professional association from the Association of Medical Superintendents of American Institutions of the Insane to the American Medico-Psychological Association in 1892, in recognition of their work's growing scientific basis. In 1922 their association was renamed again to become the current American Psychiatric Association (APA), and the profession of "psychiatry" was distinctly recognized. It was still the case, however, that practitioners preferred to remove their patients from public view, and that the mentally ill remained stigmatized as "other."

As the same time that psychiatry was redefining itself, a debate was being had about the word used for the people who worked in asylums caring for patients. While often called "attendants," alienists like Cowles began to refer to "nurses" and "nursing care" in direct reference to Nightingale-type nursing. Cowles was well acquainted with such nurses: he worked closely with Linda Richards, America's "first graduate nurse," to establish a training school for nurses attached to McLean that opened in 1882.[3] The rise of professional nursing since the late 1800s had given impetus to the reform of hospital-based medicine, and the trained general nurse was seen as essential to the provision of quality inpatient care. This book explores the contemporaneous journey of nurses in psychiatry, analyzing the significance of the nursing role for the practice of psychiatry and mental health, for nursing as a profession, and for society more broadly. This is in large part an institutional history, in that the majority of psychiatric care was provided in large-scale "asylums" throughout much of the twentieth century, but it is not a story of the patient experience. Those stories have been and are being told in powerful forms in history, literature, and film,[4] and there is no doubt that psychiatric asylums, especially those run by the state, were unpleasant places, at best. Yet superintendents did at times try to make them into places of healing for poorly understood problems, and nurses were essential to that process. In this sense, this is a history of approaches to care rather than attempts to cure.

The chapters in this book do not assume that changes in psychiatric theory and ideas were applied directly and worked miracles. Indeed, many therapeutic approaches are notable for their failure and the harm they caused. As Jonathan Sadowsky has argued, it is well known that some psychiatric practices were problematic, and that they continued anyway. Our job as historians is not necessarily to reclaim those that were once effective or to discredit others, but rather to understand the complex meanings that psychiatric practices evoked and to analyze the ways in which competing ideas and practices coexisted.[5] At times, nurses were complicit in harmful approaches, and at other times there was a significant disconnect between what psychiatrists thought should happen in asylums and what nurses actually did. This book focuses on what nurses said, rather than what they actually did. It focuses on how they engaged with ideas relevant to their practice, how they "talked about therapy," how this talking led to new therapies, and how the talk about therapy was part of a program aimed at developing both knowledge and power for the profession of psychiatric nursing. The significance of nursing in psychiatry relates to the idea of *care*, so this book focuses on the processes by which nurses struggled to develop a knowledge and practice of their own that would positively affect the work they did and the impact they had on patients. In the space created for the rise of the psychological expert, nurses took their role seriously and saw themselves as central to the reform of institutions, as well as to the broad social program of understanding, and healing, the American psyche.[6]

It was in the period immediately following World War II that psychiatric nursing was able to establish itself as the first graduate clinical specialty in nursing. But nurses had been arguing for this development for decades. This book is an analysis of the complex and sometimes contradictory dynamics of that process, and explores the knowledge and theory that nurses needed to generate in this period by which they could make claims to a unique practice. The frameworks and approaches that they developed in the mid-twentieth century drew on earlier ideas, and went on to inform not just psychiatric nursing but all of nursing more broadly, especially in the way that nurses came to think about their relationships with patients. In this exploration of the historical origins of psychiatric nursing, we can both critique and reclaim the assumptions and narratives that have come to underpin that practice today, and thereby reach a deeper understanding of what it actually means "to care" in mental health.[7]

The Problem of Mental Health

Throughout its history, approaches to mental illness have been plagued by the twin problems of vague diagnostic science and a lack of practitioners for treatment and care. In its 2015 *Behavioral Health Barometer*, the Substance Abuse and Mental Health Services Administration (SAMHSA) reported that 9.8 million adult Americans were living with a diagnosis of "Serious Mental Illness." Of these people, only 65.3 percent had actually received some kind of service for that illness.[8] In 2012 the same agency reported that 20 percent of adult Americans (45.9 million people) had experienced some form of mental illness in the past year. Of these people, 11.1 million reported an unmet need for services. SAMSHA reports detail a number of problems facing the mental health workforces, which include staff shortages, aging, high turnover, and lack of adequate compensation. SAMSHA states that mental health professional workforce shortages are so profound that at least 1,846 psychiatrists and 5,931 other practitioners are required across 77 percent of U.S. counties.[9] In May 2018 the Bureau of Labor Statistics reported a total of only 25,630 full-time psychiatrists employed across the country.[10]

Nurses represent by far the largest workforce in relation to mental health, not just in specialist facilities but across the entirety of the health spectrum. U.S. registered nurses currently number 4.1 million, with roughly 4 percent (164,000) of these nurses working in psychiatric/mental health settings.[11] Today, psychiatric mental health nurse practitioners currently number about 4.5 percent of the total registered nurse workforce, or 19,000 certified advanced practice nurses.[12] They advocate an "integrated" model of care that recognizes often complex diagnoses, multiple treatment approaches, and the social and personal situations of client across all health settings.

Integrated care also recognizes the importance of health promotion and patient-centered wellness approaches, often in community or home-based settings. This model of care is in stark contrast to that currently practiced by psychiatrists, which largely relies on the fifteen-minute "medication management" appointment. While some psychiatrists are beginning to critique this model,[13] it is in fact nurses who are often the front line of psychiatric and mental health care, and not just in specialist institutions or clinics but in all aspects of inpatient and outpatient care. In fact, it has been argued that it is nurses who are best positioned to meet people where they are, and to provide high-level complex care that does not rely solely on prescriptions.[14]

The World Health Organization proclaims mental health as a global public health priority, and stresses the urgent need for "high quality, culturally-appropriate health and social care in a timely way to promote recovery, in order for people to attain the highest possible level of health and participate fully in society and at work, free from stigmatization and discrimination."[15] This statement echoes many of the sentiments that motivated the passing of the National Mental Health Act in 1946, which provided funding for "the improvement of the mental health of the people of the United States" through a broad program aimed at "prevention, diagnosis and treatment of psychiatric disorders."[16] The Act provided for the establishment of the National Institute of Mental Health, and its first director, Robert Felix, interpreted "psychiatric disorders" in their broadest sense, arguing that the philosophy guiding the institute would be the belief "that prevention of mental illness, and the production of positive mental health, is an attainable goal."[17]

In the more than seventy intervening years since the passing of the National Mental Health Act, much has been written about the success or failure of the national approach to mental health and its various health professional workforces.[18] This is not a linear narrative of unalloyed progress, rather the story of mental health in the United States in the twentieth century is one of cycles of optimism and attempts at reform, followed by periods of poor funding and failures of political will. Within these cycles, psychiatric and psychological professionals became an integral part of American health care and culture.[19] In this context, science and medicine came to play important cultural and political roles as the quest for answers to social problems became more pressing. Nurses were considered part of this program: they had shown themselves to be vital to the war effort, and were now considered a central part of the American health care system, with access to patients in hospitals, clinics, communities, and homes. General nursing was a powerful profession, governed by the twin arms of the American Nurses Association (ANA) and the National League for Nursing Education. These two organizations were responsible for all of nursing's education and practice standards—except for psychiatry. By focusing on the development of general nursing within medical hospitals in the first half of the twentieth century, nursing's professional bodies were not yet equipped to deal with the issue of specialization.

The education and practice standards for work in psychiatric hospitals were largely under the control of the APA through its Central Inspection Board and its Committee on Standards and Policies.[20] By 1956 this was no longer the case. Nursing organizations had developed curriculums, standards of practice, statements on mental health, and accreditation of courses, and nurses were directors of both training schools and psychiatric hospital nursing programs. This was not an overnight process, and it is not the case that nursing ignored this issue until World War II. Rather, debates about the relationship between psychiatric nursing and general nursing were as old as trained nursing itself. There were many nurses who were concerned about psychiatric issues and psychiatric patients, but the reality of funding, education and hospital structures, and psychiatry's own ideas about asylum staff, meant that for nurses to gain control took time, and careful negotiation. Chapters 1 and 2 explore this longer history.

These negotiations often exposed a set of seemingly binary contradictions, overlaid with relationships of race and class and gender. These were contradictions between medicine and psychiatry, as well as conflicts between psychiatrists and nurses. There were conflicts between ideas of cure and care, prevention and treatment, environment and individual, control and autonomy; and conflicts within psychiatry between theory and practice, therapy and restraint, science and the social. Yet no single group, or even individual, inhabited only one position. Rather, these relationships operated as a continual dialogue and conversation along the spectrum between these extremes. Positions were changed, shared, reversed, tried out, and rejected. The significance of these binaries lies in the conversations, in what was being said and who was doing the talking. These conversations reflect the rapidly changing terrain in approaches to mental health, and they demonstrate that progress was neither linear nor inevitable, and that psychiatrists themselves were not unified and had no clear consensus on ways to proceed. These debates and ideas in nursing organizations and literature are the subject of chapters 3–5, which chart continuities and disruptions in thinking across time and place. These three chapters all have a common theme—that talk about psychiatry, its theory and method, and contests over knowledge and power always demonstrate the contingent and socially constructed nature of mental health, which is repeatedly conceptualized as a social issue as much as a medical one.[21]

Psychiatry as a Social Project

When the National Institute of Mental Health was founded in 1948, it recognized that the education and training of skilled personnel was essential to the goal of mental health, which was now conceived as much as a broad social project as an issue of individual illness. Mental health professionals expressed this view explicitly in their work; sociologists, psychologists and psychiatrists were all suddenly experts in the diagnosis and treatment of a sick society.[22] In a speech at the ANA annual convention in New Jersey in 1958, psychiatric nurse Hildegard Peplau stated that "nurses outside of psychiatric hospitals have become aware of mental illness, not only as a major health problem, but as the number one social problem of our times."[23] In this speech, and in her other work, Peplau stressed the central role of the nurse in addressing the nation's mental health needs, which she saw as inherently social. It was this statement from Peplau that sparked my interest in the broader cultural and political context of the role of the nurse in American psychiatry and mental health, in which mental illness was conceived as a "social problem" and indeed the greatest social problem of the time.

The federal appropriation of funds after World War II signaled a formal commitment to the idea of mental health as more than just an individual medical problem; it articulated a program aimed at understanding and transforming human behavior.[24] As Ellen Herman, Martin Halliwell, and Michael Staub argue, this process began before World War II, when many U.S. psychologists, psychiatrists, and social theorists were engaged in theoretical and clinical studies aimed at understanding the collective nature of fascism and authoritarianism.[25] The concern with the social context of mental illness had a longer history in the mental hygiene movement, which had suggested that illness could be linked to, and prevented by, social conditions.[26] From the 1930s, the psychiatric approach included a more overt and particularly "American" engagement with Freud, in that it was characterized less by interest in the sexual elements of

Freudian theory and more in the social effects of repression, sublimation, and the death drives.[27] In particular, Freud's post-World War I work attributed potential social origins to both individual and collective behavior. These ideas found purchase in American psychological and psychiatric thought from the 1930s onward in the context of another impending world war and facilitated the growth of what was sometimes loosely referred to as "social psychiatry."[28] This was a psychiatry aimed at a whole society: mental health practitioners, policy makers, and government all sought to uncover the social origins of mental illness and its link to all forms of social disturbance.

It was psychiatry's role in war in particular that helped to legitimize it as a profession that was now authorized to make claims akin to the social sciences.[29] As a discipline, psychiatry appeared to offer answers to complex problems of individual and social pathology, and a means of understanding the enemy abroad and at home. It provided treatment tools, theories, and research methodologies that could be used to study, understand, and hopefully control, human behavior.[30] The nature and consequences of two world wars led to the "socialization" of psychiatry on a multitude of fronts. Initially the concern was with repatriation and demobilization, specifically how to integrate soldiers (not just the wounded and traumatized but the mentally healthy as well) back into the day-to-day reality of postwar life. For the wounded (physically, mentally, and often both), there were concerns with access to and the quality of care, as well as with family acceptance and workplace productivity. The men had changed, but society had shifted as well, so adjustment would need to be a collective effort.

Deborah Weinstein and Anna Creadick have demonstrated how these tensions led to psychiatry's infiltration into the heart of the American family as a central component of social stability.[31] Such social stability rested on a particular kind of "normal" defined by adherence to gender, class, and race role stereotypes; disciplined productivity; a sound mind and body; and commitment to democratic ideals.[32] Yet after World War II in particular, the reality of American life was itself the biggest threat to social stability. While Americans were being exhorted to adjust, adapt, and be happy, they were simultaneously exposed to the paranoia and hysteria of anticommunist (and anti-homosexual) McCarthyism, the horrors of the bombings of Hiroshima and Nagasaki, and the descent into a nuclear-fueled Cold War.[33] Women who had thrived in war work were now being told to return to traditional roles. The hypocrisy of segregated army units and anger over the inequitable treatment of Black soldiers highlighted the long term consequences of the devastation of Jim Crow and threatened to shake society to the core.

Halliwell has argued that the mid-twentieth century saw an increasing med-
icalization of everyday life and the emergence of a whole-scale "therapeutic
culture" in which the fear that society was inherently sick existed alongside the
belief that society could and should be cured.[34] This dual belief, Halliwell
argues, fueled the "emphasis on science and medicine during the Cold War,"
which is "central to understanding the direction of state-sponsored research,
university funding, and laboratory projects."[35] It is in this pervading sociocul-
tural context that large sums of money were appropriated for the development
of the mental health professions. Social workers, psychologists, psychiatrists,
and nurses all jockeyed for position, sometimes as colleagues and sometimes
as rivals. Ultimately, these professions needed to find ways to work together,
and, in doing so, they challenged long-held beliefs about mental health and illness, and the role of women in the care of the sick.

Nurses in the History of Psychiatry

While it is the case that psychiatry in the twentieth century was an overtly
"social" project, and that this context informed the development of nursing practice, it is also the case that nurses were more immediately concerned with the
individual therapeutic effect of their work. They hoped to inform social understandings, but their day-to-day work was concerned with the conditions of
patient care, the intimacies and struggles of life in an asylum, and the small tasks
that consumed nurses' working lives. This focus on care has been both boon
and burden to nurses throughout their history. For many, care is the essence of
nursing practice, but the difficulty of defining what care means, and the historically gendered assumptions that accompany definitions of care, have complicated how nurses have been seen throughout history.[36] The focus of scholarship
on the history of psychiatry is often on the endeavors of white male psychiatrists and their "big" ideas, and this has been both a consequence of and con-
tributor to the invisibility of nurses in the history of psychiatry. The story of
two historical documents is illustrative of some of the dynamics present in this
relationship between cure and care, which has come to affect the way that psychiatric history has been written.

In 1952 the APA published the first *Diagnostic and Statistical Manual:
Mental Disorders* (more commonly known as the DSM-I). Since 1918 the APA
had drawn on the classificatory work of Emil Kraepelin[37] to construct the *Statistical Manual for the Use of Institutions for the Insane*.[38] This document had
proven inadequate for the use of military psychiatry during World War II, and
was revised by the APA's Statistics and Nomenclature Committee in 1948. This
committee included psychiatrists Harry Stack Sullivan and William Menninger,

who had lead the U.S. Army's Selective Service and Neuropsychiatry Divisions. DSM-I divided mental illness into two large groupings, one based on classifications related to impairment of brain function and the other comprising the more neurotic or psychotic problems of adjustment.[39] As Albert Deutsch explained in 1962, the problem with Kraepelin's work had been his inability to articulate "why" mental illness occurred. Deutsch's concern with etiology was central to DSM-I and reflected a significant shift in American psychiatry toward psychodynamic and psychoanalytic theories. The effect of DSM-I was profound, and, as a "scientific" document, it solidified psychiatry's place in American medicine, politics, and culture. It became the immediate requisite document for institutional classification and treatment of patients, and did so in such a way that psychiatrists, superintendents, and medical students were forced to consider the environmental and social nature of mental illness.[40]

The other historical document is a book published in 1952 by Hildegard Peplau, then an assistant professor at Teachers College, Columbia University. Titled *Interpersonal Relations in Nursing: A Conceptual Frame of Reference for Psychodynamic Nursing*, the book was the result of many years of study and practical experience. As a nurse and a student, Peplau had long been concerned with the psychoanalytic and psychodynamic aspects of the nursing role in psychiatry, and she brought an impressive depth of experience to her translation of psychological theory for nursing practice. Peplau had earned a degree in interpersonal psychology from Bennington College in Vermont, where she had studied with Erich Fromm and Harry Stack Sullivan. She had undertaken placements at the prestigious psychoanalytic-focused inpatient treatment center Chestnut Lodge, in Maryland, where she had worked intensively with Frida Fromm-Reichmann. Peplau had served at the 312th Field Hospital for Military Neuropsychiatry in England during World War II, where she worked directly with William Menninger, who offered her a job in Topeka, Kansas, after the war. She was certified as a psychoanalyst at the William Alanson White Institute in New York City, where she regularly studied and talked with Harry Stack Sullivan, Karen Horney, and Frieda Fromm-Reichmann.[41] Yet when Peplau sought a publisher for her dissertation on psychodynamic nursing, which was actually completed in 1948, she struggled to establish her legitimacy. Publishers saw the importance of her work, but repeatedly asked, "Wouldn't you rather publish this with a physician?" No, said Miss Peplau, she would not.[42] In the context of an educational environment in which all of the psychiatric nursing textbooks were written by psychiatrists (most of whom were superintendents of asylums), it took four years of being a faculty member at Teachers College before Peplau could convince a press to publish her work. As we will see in chapter 1,

psychiatrists themselves understood how important nurses were to the transformation of patient care, and advocated for the development of advanced nursing schools and the active participation of the nurse in the therapeutic team.
Yet nurses continually struggled to have their voices heard, and are largely
absent from the story of psychiatry in American history.

Historian Gerald Grob has argued that during the extensive reform and
revival of the mental health professions in the early twentieth century nurses
were near the bottom of the prevailing hierarchies due to high workforce attrition and a lack of scholarship.[43] The purpose of this book is not to prove
Grob wrong, but rather to argue for a more nuanced understanding of the role
of the nurse in the history of psychiatric care, and to situate the development of
the nursing profession in its social and historical context. There is much to
learn about the transformation of psychiatric theory and practice in the twentieth century through the lens of the nurse. Historian John Burnham has argued
that the tumult surrounding the psychological professions in the first half of
the twentieth century opened up space for innovation in theory and practice,
and that "paramedical" personnel such as nurses were essential to this process.[44] However, despite a large body of work that traces the effects of war on the
health service professions, explores attempts at institutional reform, charts the
move to community-based services, and studies the impact of psychotropic drugs
and the antipsychiatry movement, historians have not generally considered the
role of professional nursing in these systems.[45]

Similarly, within a rapidly expanding field of nursing history scholarship,
the significance of the development of psychiatric nursing in the United States
has not been the subject of extensive inquiry. The work that does exist tends to
focus on the key stages of the development of the profession or its related associations.[46] Some historians have attempted to trace the legacy of Peplau as the
key figure in the history of psychiatric nursing. Barbara Callaway has written
an intricate and detailed biography, and Tom Olson has endeavored to explore
the significance of Peplau's theory of interpersonal relations in the mid-twentieth
century.[47] Olson has argued that this was an important, but difficult, time for
American nurses as they struggled to identify what was unique to their practice
and debated the place of mental health nursing as a specialty in nurse education. For Olson, the problem for mental health nursing lay in its reliance on
interpersonal theory, which he believes was "unstable" ground on which to
build the profession given the rapid advance of pharmacological therapies. However, D'Antonio and colleagues have argued that challenges facing psychiatric
nursing today are not due to any inherent weakness in the theory of interpersonal relations but rather to "the biologically and specialty based imperatives

that have subsumed the significance of relationships in our practice."[48] They argue that there is much to be learnt from mid-century psychiatric nurse theorists like Peplau, who championed the idea of the therapeutic relationship as the essence of *all* nursing practice.[49] They demonstrate that Peplau's theory was grounded in her social context, and was designed to make a specific contribution to a democratic social effort.[50] This was an idea that required nurses to make the most of emerging funding opportunities, but it also required them to develop new and specific knowledge in order to do so.

Peplau, however, was not the only nurse who thought this way; nor was hers the only attempt to develop psychiatric nursing into a wider social program. Indeed, many nurses prior to Peplau had seen the broader social importance of mental health work, not only through their previous engagement with mental hygiene, but also in the social context of public health nursing itself.[51] This social aspect of nursing practice—not just the recognition of the importance of nursing for the nation's health, but also a recognition of the social determinants of the health of patients, and the intersections between class, race, and health—found expression in the emergence of psychiatric nursing as a specialty, and goes beyond the work of Peplau.

Knowledge and Power in Psychiatric Nursing

On an everyday level, given the reality of physician staffing levels in institutions, it was the nursing staff who were in fact responsible for the interpretation and application of psychiatric treatment.[52] Paramedical personnel like nurses have also been referred to as "intermediaries" by Ryan Johnson and Amna Khalid, who argue that bringing a Subaltern Studies approach to an analysis of the role of those traditionally considered subordinate in health care systems can demonstrate the way that "colonial policy was not a top-down process but one that subordinates and intermediaries helped to negotiate and shape."[53] This is especially true in the colonial setting, where those at the periphery enact the demands of the center, but in ways that are altered by both the subjectivity of the intermediaries themselves and the reality of the colonial situation. The role of nurses as intermediaries has been explored in various aspects of nursing and public health history, especially in relation to colonial territories and diasporas, and in contexts where women negotiate multiple subjectivities as nurses, workers, and minorities.[54] The limited existing histories of mental health nursing also argue that mental health work and the people who do it have been shaped by a number of intersecting forces, including changing notions of respectable work for women, shifts in ideas about care and treatment in psychiatry, and the changing social and political contexts of approaches to mental health.[55]

Important work on the role of the nurse in the development of new psychiatric treatment approaches in Europe has revealed that nurses were often as complicit in traumatizing treatments as they were in advocating for more humane approaches to patient care, and this reflects the multiple social and political factors that nurses needed to negotiate in that time and place.[56] As psychiatry itself has been seen as a force for both good and evil in the world, so too have psychiatric nurses.

Social control is never too far from discussions of psychiatric history, and in this history we can see the way in which ideas that we now take for granted in mental health originated from a particular social moment in a particular political context. Throughout the first half of the twentieth century, ideas about mental health and illness were as strongly linked to the ideology of American "freedom" as they were to an idea of what constituted "normal" personhood. This tendency toward categorization and normalization, which then allowed for the treatment, institutionalization, and sometimes incarceration of the different, was the backbone of the antipsychiatry critique. Michel Foucault argued that psychiatric mental health professions cannot be separated from the state's use of biopower to create disciplined minds and bodies.[57] This includes bodies of color, who are noticeably absent from the dominant narrative of psychiatric nursing practice. Nursing was a racially segregated profession for the first half of the twentieth century, as were psychiatric institutions. Psychiatry itself has been accused of being a racially charged practice, in which deliberate decisions about diagnosis and treatment were historically linked to the attempts to stifle and criminalize those involved in civil rights movements.[58] A study of the role of African American nurses' involvement in psychiatry is the subject of chapter 5, and provides a critical analysis of the complex ways in which the complexities of race for mental health were negotiated, or ignored, by nursing.

Psychiatric nurses were, and still are, implicated in these social processes, either as intermediaries, negotiators, resistors, or perpetrators. This is not an idea that nursing scholars today have shied away from. Indeed, nurse philosophers seek explicitly to engage with the tensions at the heart of mental health nursing practice through Foucault's theory of governmentality and recognition of the inherent power of psychiatry to control or influence people's minds.[59] If we were to consider asylums the center of psychiatric colonization, then nurses and other institutional staff become the lens through which to explore the reality of that process. Their experiences, rendered through their subjectivity or sense of self as women, as nurses, and as workers, demonstrate the contingent nature of psychiatric practice, and the mediation of psychiatric treatment ideas by the practical reality of the institution.

Dave Holmes, Denise Gastaldo, Amelie Perron, Trudy Rudge, and Thomas Foth, among others, all argue that mental health nursing has a history and is a practice fraught with contradiction.[60] These contradictions provide the framework for this book: the desire to "help" against the effect of control; the ideal of theory against the reality of practice; the social problem against the individual solution; and the scientific center against the subjectivity of the periphery. The chapters that follow seek to demonstrate that the particular social and political circumstances surrounding ideas about mental health in the early to mid-twentieth century facilitated the development of psychiatric nursing in a particular time and place, and determined the course that it would take. Psychiatric nurses engaged with prevailing ideas and the surrounding political environment in ways that have come to underpin contemporary nursing practice, and which established psychiatric and mental health nursing as a distinctly white woman's knowledge project.[61]

Chapter 1

"The Backbone of Every Mental Hospital"

Defining Nursing in Early Psychiatry

For as long as there have been specialist institutions for the mentally ill there have been debates about who should work in them, and what that work should look like. During the late nineteenth century, the management philosophies of asylums shifted from custodial to medical, with an increasing public and policy expectation that asylums would be places of actual treatment and care. At the same time, the growth of asylum populations meant that superintendents increasingly "managed at a remove,"[1] which placed pressure on the existing workforce, and gave rise to a reassessment of the role of the nurse. The rise of modern "trained nursing" and the development of nursing schools had transformed general hospitals, and psychiatrists began to look to nurses to do the same for asylums, both because they were trained and because they were women. While nurses themselves were active in creating their approach to psychiatric work, it was both with and against psychiatrists' points of view that nurses came to imagine, and then make, themselves.

The relationship between psychiatry and nursing in the early part of the twentieth century lay the groundwork for the emergence of psychiatric nursing as an advanced clinical specialty, and established the patterns of both cooperation and conflict between the two professions. Psychiatrists, particularly through the American Psychiatric Association (APA),[2] agitated for trained nurses to become their main workforce, and actively worked to reform their education and training. In analyzing this reform process, we can see the ways in which ideas about nurses' "essential nature" as women were central to arguments for their use in asylums. These gendered ideas existed at the same time as psychiatrists expressed a need for the trained nurses' real skill and knowledge, and it was this need that became the impetus for the development of advanced educa-tion over which the APA believed it should have control. Ironically, however, in initiating a formal attempt to prescribe and define psychiatric nursing, the APA set in motion the process that would end its very ability to do so.

While nurses themselves were only a small proportion of the workforce in institutions, they rose to the top of the inpatient care-providing hierarchy as a result of a long process of negotiation, consultation, and conflict with profes-sional psychiatry, particularly the APA. Since its origins, the APA had formally controlled the standards for practice and education that nurses working in psy-chiatric institutions followed. This was not true in other areas of nursing, which had been responsible for their own accreditation and curriculums since the late 1800s. The inability of professional nursing bodies to integrate psychiatry into the new schools of nursing and the urgency of the demand for asylum pro-fessionals created a space in which the APA felt that it had the right and the mandate to control the standards and education of another profession, which it believed "belonged" to them.

For psychiatrists, the issue was largely one of legitimacy. In much the same way that physicians and surgeons had been, institutional psychiatrists were dependent on nursing staff to ensure patient health, well-being, and recovery, ultimately influencing the reputation of psychiatry itself. And in the same way that medical hospital managers had, psychiatric hospital administrators real-ized that education and training of staff was the key to their success. The legiti-macy of the emerging profession of psychiatry rested on its ability to be taken seriously as both a medical and scientific practice.[3] This would require that asy-lums be serious places of treatment and care, more than mere institutions of custodial containment. The central concern of psychiatrists to move toward therapeutic treatment and care was the starting point for the reform of related institutional workforces, especially in nursing.

The Origins of Specialty Psychiatric Care

Following the reforms set in motion by Philippe Pinel in France in the late 1700s, the establishment of small asylums such as the York Retreat in the United Kingdom in 1796 and the Friends Asylum in Pennsylvania in 1813 had brought into sharp relief the nature of the care provided by asylum staff.[4] Small asylums were more able to initiate programs that reflected more directly the philosophy of the superintendent, which from the early 1800s included the desire to move away from restraint as a mode of care and an emphasis on "moral treatment."[5] Moral treatment may have worked well in small asylums, especially those estab-lished by Quakers, where relationships were based on reciprocal arrangements between families and communities and where inmates cared for each other through various stages of recovery and progressive freedoms.[6] However, as asylums grew in acceptability and accessibility, so did the need for externally acquired personnel. As psychiatrist and asylum superintendent Edward Cowles recounted in his review of the first fifty years of the APA, "The problem of the nursing of the insane arose with Pinel";[7] that is, if patients were to be released from restraints, then how else was their behavior to be managed? The concern was not just about reducing the risks of patients' harm to themselves or others but also about affecting actual therapeutic outcomes, including potential recovery. Once asylums were established in the United States, they quickly outgrew their patient capacity, often leading to overcrowding. This tended to shift the treatment focus away from individual therapy to a collective management of people, and this required more staff.[8] However, it was not enough that staff be able to manage large groups, although this was important. It was also essential to psychiatrists that their institutions be places of perceived and actual treatment. If recovery of some sort, rather than mere custody, was the aim, psychiatrists needed to turn their attention to questions of what constituted the best kind of asylum staff to bring this about, and what sort of education and training such a staffing body would need. This would require the employment of highly skilled, trained personnel. Recognizing this need, new asylums being built along the Kirkbride model, which emphasized more open spaces and progressive patient freedoms, included plans for "the systematic instruction of attendants."[9] But it was the emergence of professional nursing that had the biggest impact on the thinking of asylum superintendents.

In 1882 Cowles had worked closely with Linda Richards, America's "first trained nurse,"[10] to establish the McLean Hospital School of Nursing in Waverly, Massachusetts. Ten years later he claimed that there were nineteen such schools and credited nursing with their establishment. He argued that it had been Florence Nightingale's reform of general hospitals and the establishment of nurse training schools that had inspired "alienists" to reform their own institutions, and that the example set by general nursing promised "a revolution in work for the insane."[11] He saw great hope for physicians and patients alike in the model being established by the new nursing schools: "This movement is filled with the largest promise of good to come by the multiplied power and inspiration it brings to physician and nurse; and it is big with blessings to the sick in mind who, even in their weakness, may know and be uplifted by the intelligent and sympathetic interest of those in whose care they are."[12] In his own school and hospital he argued that nurses formed an essential part of both the therapeutic and research programs. He counted trained nurses as essential in his quest for a more thoroughly scientific approach to understanding mental illness, and for the betterment of patient experiences and outcomes. "A great contribution to these remedial influences," he wrote in 1898, "is the introduction of the system of training nurses in our hospitals. . . . Our educated nurses have come to be actual assistants in the professional work, aiding us in clinical observations and applying for us, as was never done before, some of the most effective of our therapeutic methods."[13] Cowles made it clear that nurses were part of the "whole" team, and that their notes and observations rated with those of the physician for understanding the patient and developing care plans.

Gender in Early Psychiatric Nursing

While Cowles advocated for the development of fully trained nurses as asylum staff, he also advocated that these staff members be women. In the advertisement for applications to work at McLean, it was very clearly stated that women were sought and that, as such, they should be "sober, honest, trustworthy, punctual, quiet, orderly, cleanly, neat, patient, kind and cheerful."[14] Cowles was not the only psychiatrist to consider these important qualities for nursing staff. In the late nineteenth and early twentieth centuries a number of physicians articulated the various ways in which women nurses could contribute to patient care. A. B. Richardson, the superintendent of the Government Hospital for the Insane in Washington, DC (which would come to be known as St. Elizabeths Hospital), wrote that his program of employing women as nurses was having a marked effect on both the daily management of the hospital and on patient outcomes.[15] While Richardson did maintain an employment process for unskilled attendants, and stated that he thought there would always be a place for male attendants in asylums for heavy lifting and in case of violence, he clearly differentiated between attendants and trained nurses. In 1902 he boasted a workforce that included fifty-two graduate nurses.[16] In either case it was women as "head nurses" who had "general charge of the entire hospital service in all the wards for the acute and chronic sick and for many of the feeble classes," and on at least eight other wards they were responsible "for the nursing care of the patients, the recording of notes and the administration of remedies."[17]

Unlike general hospitals, mental hospitals were still "segregated" along gender lines; that is, female nurses or attendants were not generally permitted to work on male wards. Richardson did employ female nurses on male wards, and reported significant improvements in care and behavior—largely, he claimed, by virtue of the women's gender. He drew on many familiar tropes about the natural ability of women to nurse, arguing that women, especially through their capacity to be mothers, were naturally suited to nursing work. "They have a kinder and more sympathetic manner," he argued, and "are more patient and long suffering. Their touch is gentler."[18] In his view, these were the qualities that had made female nursing in general hospitals so successful.

Like many of his contemporaries, especially male physicians, Richardson conflated good nursing with gender stereotypes, and related the effect on patient behavior to these same social norms. For example, his male patients were more respectful to the female nurses not necessarily because of their skill but because they were women. "Men who abuse their doctors and are generally suspicious of their surroundings, often yield unquestioning obedience to the female nurse," he noted. Because of this effect, Richardson intended to expand on his program of employing women, arguing that "the introduction of one or two discreet, intelligent and trained female nurses into each ward, more particularly for the moral treatment of the patients and the general supervision of their medical treatment, is of decided advantage and entirely feasible."[19]

While all hospitals employed men, and did sometimes call them nurses, men were more frequently referred to as attendants, and their role, and the perception of their abilities, was markedly different from what psychiatrists were hoping to achieve through the shift to trained nurses.[20] Superintendents and psychiatrists drew on the standard early twentieth-century imagery of the nurse as the embodiment of womanly virtue to articulate their benefit for asylums and for patients. As early as 1906, Charles Bancroft, superintendent of the New Hampshire State Hospital, extolled the benefits of nurses for asylums on account of women's perceived natural tendencies toward tidiness, their moral influence—especially over men—and their innate homemaking skills.[21]

Bancroft also went so far as to say that he believed all wards of the institution should be under the care of a graduate nurse, and by this he meant women who had graduated from general schools of nursing, had worked in general hospitals or private duty, and had then come to asylum work bringing that wealth of experience, maturity, and intelligence. "A most important feature is the management of this entire building," he wrote, "which should be vested in a head nurse of experience."[22] He made it clear that he was arguing for women when he argued that "this should not be divided management, partly male and female. The hospital building should be absolutely under the care of the head nurse and her assistants. The nurses should feel that they are in control. Division of responsibility between male and female attendants is not productive of good results but leads rather to friction and irritation."[23] In his appeal to the psychiatric profession to pay more attention to the nature of the institutional workforce, Bancroft signaled an awareness of the growing power of professional nursing and its link to medical legitimacy, and was keenly aware that the favorable public perception of general nursing and the reform of hospitals could be used to build the respectability of psychiatry. Superintendents like Cowles, Richardson, and Bancroft were all keen to establish their practice and institutions as scientific and successful, and trained nurses were imagined as central to this process.

Beyond public relations were more mundane, practical reasons why female trained nurses were preferred for modern psychiatric institutions. At the same time as Superintendent Richardson drew on gendered rhetoric regarding the nature of the female nurse, he also made important observations about the prevailing social and economic structures that contributed to the female nurse's advantages as a worker. While their gender may have predisposed nurses to be more sympathetic, kind, and gentle in the work of caring for the insane, it was their attitude toward work itself that Richardson argued made them more valuable employees. Unlike men who sometimes came into nursing as a temporary step along their career, women, who were well aware of their limited opportunities elsewhere, saw nursing as one of the few paths open to them toward independence, autonomy, and professional satisfaction. "Women . . . are more inclined to see the work of nursing as deserving their best efforts. They take more pride in it," Richardson noted, at the same time acknowledging that "to the class from which they are chosen there are few occupations that offer more financial inducements and they are therefore, less inclined to change. They are more ready to undertake the training required because they see in the work a permanent employment at good wages."[24] Good wages of course were relative. In all cases, female nurses were paid less than men. This discrepancy made it relatively easy for superintendents to prefer training women as nurses because they could consistently pay them less. At St. Elizabeths, for example, female nurses, even when employed as head nurses, earned $30 per month, compared to the $35 per month earned by untrained male workers in the same position. Women who worked as graduate head nurses on male wards earned an extra $2.50 a month for their efforts.[25]

While there is no reason to assume that psychiatrists did not believe that women were more gentle, or kind, or naturally suited to the work of caring, it was also the case that employing women created a cheaper and more stable workforce. At the same time, drawing on the image of the trained nurse as a professional helped to negate moral fears about the exposure of young women to the notoriously inappropriate behavior of asylum inmates, and thus imbued asylums with a veneer of respectability and safety in the public eye. Psychiatrists wanted women as trained nurses because they knew trained nurses were suited for the work and produced significant improvements in patient outcomes, but also because their female presence in an institution indicated a safe, respectable, and scientific place to receive care.

The structural and economic reality of life for single middle-class women in the late nineteenth and early twentieth centuries did not deliver hordes of young women eager to embrace working in psychiatric institutions. Part of the issue, despite psychiatrists' reports to the contrary, was that training programs in general nursing (as opposed to psychiatric) remained a more attractive option to women looking to be nurses, because those programs led to registration with agencies that could find them private duty work, and qualified them for work in general hospitals. The lack of psychiatric content in the general nursing curriculum and, as Elizabeth Lunbeck has summarized, the "bureaucratic wrangling over costs and organization between hospitals and the state,"[26] meant that psychiatrists opted to establish their own training schools. They then needed to attract women to attend them, but the difficulty of doing so was both cause and effect of the continued conflict between general and specialist nursing, and between professional nursing and professional psychiatry.

The Committee on Psychiatric Nursing

The early twentieth century saw psychiatrists seek to expand the scientific basis of their profession and to align themselves more clearly with academic medicine. This move was intended to shift the perception that psychiatrists were merely custodial superintendents and promote the growing belief that mental illness was a disease like any other. Nurses therefore were essential to its treatment, but they were not easy to find. Bancroft admitted that women were less likely to make asylum nursing their first choice because "the character of the disease does not appeal to the ordinary individual,"[27] and because there was actually less demand for psychiatric nursing than general nursing. General nursing was a more stable choice for a young woman looking to commit years to furthering her education, as it opened up more opportunities than did specialized asylum training alone. He also acknowledged the public perception that lingered in assessments of the asylum nurse compared to the general nurse: "The public, as well as the nurses themselves often have the feeling that the asylum nurse does not have quite the same qualifications as her sister trained in the general hospital."[28]

This "feeling" was not without a basis in fact, and had been recognized for some time. In the establishment of the McLean Asylum Training School, Cowles and Richards had worked out a program whereby nurses who graduated from it could be admitted "under certain restrictions" to the Boston Training School for Nurses at the Massachusetts General Hospital, and after successfully completing one year's extra study would be awarded their general nursing diploma in addition to that awarded by the McLean Asylum Training School.[29] This was a rare model, however, with many general schools of nursing insisting that a full two years be dedicated to the general nursing diploma. This was an unrealistic expectation; as Bancroft noted, "The majority of nurses do not feel that they can afford the time necessary for courses of instruction in two hospitals."[30]

By the time Bancroft was thinking about the problem some fifteen years after Cowles had, the issue of this relationship between general and psychiatric nursing had not been resolved. In some ways the difference had intensified as psychiatrists became clearer about the nature of the work they wanted nurses to undertake in their asylums, which was markedly different to the work that general nursing prepared them for. Bancroft argued that general nursing education and practice was actually unsuitable for asylum work and that general nursing bred "physicians helpers," women who were used to following instructions in uncomplicated situations, where no intellectual or emotional engagement from the nurse herself was required. Bancroft's argument is interesting because he indicates the expectation that nurses will be actively involved in the therapeutic program, and are not intended as mere sick nurses caring for surgical or unwell patients. "The nurse in an asylum," he stated, "is constantly being taught that the patient's judgment and responsibility are impaired and that her own judgment must ever be tactfully substituted for that of the patient. Tact and self-control become cardinal virtues in the asylum nurse. . . . Most general hospital nurses, undertaking special training in an asylum, become impatient, see nothing to do and grow weary under the constant demands made upon their nervous energy."[31] In Bancroft's scenario psychiatric nursing was being conceptualized as an active therapeutic practice, where the work was emotional and required the nurse to "be with" as opposed to "do to" the patient. This was a markedly different theory and philosophy of nursing than that being generated in general nursing, and would in fact become the basis of arguments within nursing itself in years to come.[32] While Bancroft later suggested that graduate nurses who had general experience and then came to work in asylums were capable of this way of working, and were highly valued because of it, he acknowledged that this pathway was rare. In lieu of this pattern, and given the lack of psychiatric content in the general nursing curriculum, psychiatrists moved to formalize the training of their own staff.

Bancroft was appointed chair of a subcommittee of the APA dedicated to the articulation of standards for training schools for nurses, and it released its first statement of ideas in the July 1906 issue of the *American Journal of Psychiatry*.[33]

The subcommittee members included four other psychiatrists—Charles Clarke, Arthur Hurd, William Russell, and George Tuttle—and mentioned that some input had been received from nurses who were superintendents of nurse training schools in hospitals of the insane: Mary May, Marie Ferrier, Sara Parsons, Linda Richards, and Lucia Woodward.[34] There was no formal consultation at this stage with the new official nursing organizations such as the Nurses Associated Alumnae (precursor of the American Nurses Association) or the American Society of Superintendents of Training Schools for Nurses (later the National League for Nursing Education).[35] While the APA was aware that these organizations existed, the fact that they were not in formal consultation at this stage speaks to the still emerging nature of those organizations, and the APA's belief that it knew what was best for nursing.

The APA subcommittee report therefore made comprehensive recommendations across all aspects of establishing and running a training school for nurses, including a potential schedule of courses over either a two- or even three-year program. Bancroft acknowledged that he adapted a large part of the material from the existing "Outline of Practical Training" from the New York State Hospital (which had a training school for nurses), where committee member William Russell was the superintendent. While the report suggested that the superintendent of all nurse training schools should be a nurse, it was noted that "the Superintendent of the Hospital will probably avoid trouble by educating one of his own nurses for this position."[36] The actual learning material would come from physicians and the course content was largely medically or sick-nursing focused, with only two courses that seemed specific to psychiatric theory or practice: "Physical Therapeutics" (spread over two semesters as "Massage & Elementary Gymnastics" and "Hydrotherapy & Application of Electricity") and "Psychology, Nervous Diseases and Insanity." The programs were imagined as either two- or three-year models because they were in fact attempting to teach general nursing principles with some overlay with psychiatric work; that is, how general nursing principles play out in psychiatric patients. Herein lay the problem: asylums needed nurses who were generally trained to care for sick people, but in the specific context of psychiatric problems, and they also needed to know about treatments for psychiatric illness itself. This was not a problem that could be solved in the lead-up to World War I, which drained the country of its nursing resources, and the approach to training schools remained sporadic and ad hoc.

After World War I, the APA picked up the issue again when it formalized its approach to psychiatric nursing in 1918. The Committee on Nursing established itself as a formal standing subcommittee of the APA and recognized that "from the standpoint of the care of patients the backbone of every mental hospital is the nursing body—that the physician's efforts could bear fruit only if carried out and supplemented by a staff of intelligent, sympathetic and interested nurses."[37] Picking up on the findings of the earlier report, this committee began to more systematically document and evaluate the standards of training schools within existing psychiatric institutions. In 1921 the committee undertook a survey of 183 state and private mental hospitals that revealed the sporadic and uncoordinated approach to the issue of nurse education. For example, only seventy-two of the hospitals surveyed had training schools at all (sixty-six of them being in state hospitals); there was no standard length or type of course; and only forty-eight of the total schools met state requirements for affiliation with general hospitals, which reduced dramatically the opportunity for general nurses to undertake any psychiatric training.

The APA considered a good course length to be two or three years, as this was what was expected in general nursing, and only 26 percent of mental hospitals maintained courses of this length.[38] Superintendents largely reported that they faced difficulties in attracting students, in arranging for affiliations with general hospitals, and in maintaining schools at all. The committee felt that the time was ripe to actively move forward in this area, that psychiatry had made considerable progress as a socially acceptable form of "medicine" in the first quarter of the twentieth century, and that higher expectations of institutions in relation to patient outcomes meant that "proper nursing care of the mentally ill" was central to the future of the profession. Superintendents themselves put the responsibility for action back on the APA. As Elisha Cohoon, superintendent of Medfield State Hospital in Massachusetts and writer of the report argued, "A great majority of the superintendents felt that the association did have a very definite responsibility in regard to it [nurse education] and should take steps to discharge that responsibility."[39]

In the immediate postwar environment, the Committee on Nursing felt an extra sense of urgency in the context of growing inpatient populations. At a meeting of the APA in Quebec in June 1922, superintendents debated the many issues that faced the establishment of high-quality training for nurses. As nursing organizations began to establish their own criteria for general nursing (which still did not include psychiatry), it became harder for training schools in psychiatric institutions to meet those general nursing standards. In attempting to do so, Dr. Harris from the New York State Hospital suggested, "we attempt to give our nurses too much medicine. We are making medical students out of them in a way, and I think that it is unnecessary."[40] He did not mean that nurses should not be educated in that way, but rather that psychiatric nursing education needed more psychiatry in it.

Dr. Russell, the superintendent at Bloomingdale Hospital in New York, agreed, stating that the attempt to meet both general and psychiatric require- ments had created a situation in which "even with our own students we ought, I believe, to put more emphasis on psychiatric training. In our schools most of the systematic nurse training is along general hospital lines, and we do not give careful enough attention to developing psychiatric nurses."[41] The superinten- dents argued about the best way to achieve this. Was it through short affiliations between general and psychiatric nursing schools; was it longer, one-year courses added to general nursing; or was it standalone two- or three-year training in psychiatric hospitals? There was no easy fix, and in part this was because the psy- chiatrists were seemingly so hesitant to discuss the issue with nurses them- selves. Cohoon realized that this situation could not continue, given the growing power and status of professional nursing. He expressed his concern at the meeting in 1922 when he said, "I think it cannot be denied that at the present time the development of nursing has reached a point where its relative impor- tance is very much increased, even to that extent where the physician may be justified in hesitating to discuss a purely nursing problem."[42] It was the influ- ence of the mental hygiene movement, however, that appeared to open up a space for dialogue between nurses and psychiatrists.

The Role of the Nurse in Mental Hygiene

In 1922 Dr. Arthur Ruggles was elected chair of the APA's Committee on Nurs- ing. As the superintendent of Butler Hospital he had been responsible for the care of Clifford Beers, the founder of the mental hygiene movement, and Rug- gles brought this concern with mental hygiene to the committee (and to the APA more generally when he became president in 1942). In 1926 Ruggles made a direct overture to trained nurses. That year he published an article in the *Amer- ican Journal of Nursing* in which he set out new ideas about neurosis, psycho- sis, and the relationship between body and mind.[43] He wrote directly to nurses in this article, appealing for them to consider the importance of knowledge about the human mind for their work in general nursing, and to recognize their role in the mental hygiene movement. He made a clear argument that the mental aspects of illness could not be separated out from all nursing, stating that "the nurse who cannot understand the patient's motivation is a liability and not an asset."[44] Nurses needed to be aware of these factors of human behavior in all of their work. Ruggles felt that this could be achieved through a "broadening cultural background in the pre-nursing school years,"[45] which for him meant a more liberal arts based education, and a more mature nursing workforce. He acknowledged the growing importance of the nurse in all areas of community and social life and admitted that the expanded role of the nurse sometimes made it difficult to differentiate between other professions, such as psychiatric social work, but he clearly felt that there was a single and particular role for the nurse in both institutions and the community.

This was particularly evident in Ruggles's plea for nurses to actively engage with the mental hygiene movement, which he saw as an important social project as opposed to a cluster of symptoms isolated to institutional care: "Mental Hygiene aims to better the treatment of mental diseases, but even more important in its program is the prevention of mental disease and the increasing of human efficiency and happiness through the direction of better mental adjustments. In such a program, the nurse is an indispensable link, and without a sufficient number of psychiatric nurses, this work must necessarily be delayed, and the reduction of feeble-mindedness, poverty, delinquency, crime and mental disease be retarded. Surely this is a challenge that the nursing world will not fail to meet."[46] Ruggles drew on the pride and heritage of American public health nursing, and the patriotic nostalgia of nurses' involvement in the recent war to remind nurses that their function was social as much as medical. It was through psychiatric work conceived in its broadest social sense that this seemingly natural tendency within American nursing could be the impetus to remove the obstacles that continued to separate physical from "mental" nursing. "Mental hygiene needs you," he declared, "and mental disease and mental defect will be prevented more rapidly if you are ready to take your part in this great war against one of the enemies of human health and happiness."[47]

Ruggles was not the only psychiatrist who argued that nurses should include mental hygiene in their education and practice. At the Biennial Convention of the American Nurses Association in Kentucky in 1928, William Russell argued that now that psychiatric medicine had expanded into the social realm, and concerned itself with issues of prevention, so too should nurses. Like Ruggles, he argued that the tradition and structures of public health nursing already placed nurses in the perfect position to work with "problems related to mentality, and to the behavior of the human being as a psycho-physical organism."[48] Nurses were used to treating, and understanding, the patient as a product of their whole environment—family, cultural, socioeconomic—so to see this environment as connected to mental health and illness was a natural progression. It would, however, require special skills and knowledge. While Russell applauded the advances that Nightingale nursing had brought to general hospitals, he argued that he was yet to see this kind of effect flow through the mental hospitals, or to public health nursing, largely because of the insistence on the separation of mind and body. Modern psychiatry did not make this differentiation, and so nursing needed to include education about psychiatric concepts at all levels. If this were the case, then nurses would be able to act as both early diagnosticians and preventative forces in the home and community—educating people about the types of environments that were thought to induce mental illness, helping people deal with stress and family problems, and recognizing symptoms before they escalated.[49]

Dr. A. E. Bennett reiterated this point in his presentation to public health nurses at the State Nurses' Association Meeting of Iowa in 1928. For this physician, mental hygiene work was essential if the nurse was to be "an efficient agent in handling public health social problems."[50] In this addition of the word "social" to "public health problems," Bennett took the role of nursing out of the ward or bedside and into the realm of society more broadly. Mental hygiene, for Bennett, was aimed explicitly at understanding both individual and collective behavior that led not simply to personal mental illness but to deviant and pathological social behaviors. Bennett argued that nurses should be contributing to the aims of mental hygiene, which included "the working out of causes and prevention of delinquency, crime, mental disease and all social maladjustments."[51] Psychiatry as mental hygiene was all-pervasive, beginning at the start of life with habit formation and personal relationships, and was concerned with intelligence and academic success as much as nervousness or personality disorders. In this work "the nurse will emphasize the importance of considering proper habit-training, self-control, the study of the type of associates, spoiled-child reactions, day-dreaming, shut-in tendencies, etc."[52] Bennett's conception of the role of the nurse placed her at the center of an almost total social surveillance and disciplining project, which demanded a level of education and knowledge not common to the profession. Indeed, nurses were being left behind in this work because other professions like social work had been quick to develop specialist psychiatric training. "The public health nurse," Bennett argued, "can never properly enter this field without taking the right kind of postgraduate, psychiatric training."[53] It was time that nursing rose to the challenge and accepted its "share of the responsibility"[54] in this important social project.

Taken on its own, psychiatry's side of the story presents a narrow view of what was in reality a complex and dynamic relationship with nursing. There is plenty of evidence that psychiatrists felt strongly about the need for skilled and educated nurses, and that they attempted to put in place some structures that might make the development of psychiatric nursing as a distinct profession possible. Psychiatrists and superintendents did clearly differentiate between attendants and nurses, and they clearly felt that those nurses should be women, and not only because that was the case for general nursing. Yet while they drew on gendered tropes to describe psychiatric nursing work, the skills they actually wanted were only attainable through a thoughtful and theoretically comprehensive program of study. Psychiatrists were torn between collaborating with nurses on what seemed to be a nursing problem and the realization that to do so would mean the ultimate relinquishment of their control of another profession. They were more and more forced to work with nurses in order to improve the quality of psychiatric nursing, and as they did so they were more and more forced to cede their control over it. The changes that came to psychiatric nursing built on these early efforts of psychiatrists and nurses to work together, but also stretched the willingness of both parties to compromise.

Chapter 2

"The Gospel of Mental Hygiene"

Reimagining Practice before World War II

The mental hygiene movement began as an attempt to reform conditions in institutions, but quickly became a broader social project aimed at prevention and social reform. These were ideas that many nurses took up with enthusiasm, and they formed the basis of their argument for an increased emphasis on mental health content in nurse education and practice. Nurses argued for the usefulness of mental hygiene on many fronts: in expanding the role of the nurse into new spaces, in the improvement of patient care and conditions, and in the development of new knowledge about the workings of the brain. This was a mental hygiene conceived broadly, reflecting the dynamic and eclectic nature of psychiatric thinking in the first half of the twentieth century. It would ultimately prove a limited and problematic model, but in engaging with the concepts that underpinned the movement, mental hygiene acted as a springboard to innovations in thinking and practice that would resonate into the second half of the twentieth century.

Nurses' engagement with the concept of mental hygiene would form the basis for a complete overhaul of nurse education in mental health once funds were available after 1946. Their writings in both published journals and textbooks in the period between the two world wars frame mental hygiene as a natural extension of public health work, with new possibilities for an expanded and autonomous scope of practice. Nurses argued that mental hygiene and the idea of prevention were significant because they were seen as a way for nurses to contribute to the development of new scientific understandings of human behavior and to participate in the interwar project of restoring social stability. Nurses emphasized the importance of child and family mental health for this work. In their publications, nurses also argued that an understanding of mental health and psychiatric concepts was essential for all nursing work as they shifted theory and practice away from a focus on illness symptoms to whole patient care. In this work, nurses argued for a more complex understanding of the nature of human health and illness and debated the ways in which psychiatric concepts could be used to improve patient care across the full spectrum of nursing activities. Through mental hygiene, they engaged with changing ideas in psychiatric thinking about the nature of mental illness itself and showed a shift toward a more complex understanding of human behavior as occurring along a spectrum and influenced by environment.

At the same time as they wrote about the usefulness and desirability of mental hygiene, nurses identified a number of issues and barriers to the improvement of practice, and to the integration of psychiatric mental health concepts into nurse education. Much of this work originated from nurses associated with major inpatient facilities in the northern states, in particular the Henry Phipps Clinic at Johns Hopkins Hospital in Baltimore. Nurses such as Harriet Bailey, Effie Taylor, and May Kennedy were particularly vocal in this space, contributing to knowledge, practice, and policy for decades and influencing the next generation. In their pleas for the inclusion and reform of mental health theory and practice, these nurses highlighted significant barriers in the existing structures of training, education, and workplaces that limited the ability of mental health workers to be taken seriously, to address encroachments from other professions, and to take control for their own education and practice away from the psychiatric associations. It is also the case that in their engagement with and writing about mental hygiene, nurses revealed limits and contradictions within the theory itself that would continue to cause a tension within nursing knowledge and practice about mental health. This tension lay at the intersection between care and control—in its emphasis on prevention, mental hygiene also relied on surveillance of the patient in their total environment, and despite its liberating potential also had strong tendencies toward normalization and even eugenics. The extent to which nurses could challenge this rhetoric was limited by the political and cultural context of American life in the interwar years, and this undermined the ability of nurses to fully imagine an autonomous practice at this point. In this context, the promise of mental hygiene work would prove somewhat illusory.

Mental Hygiene as Public Health

As one of the nation's largest inpatient psychiatric hospitals, it is not surprising that St. Elizabeths in Washington, DC, would have a curriculum for nurse education, but it is perhaps surprising that mental hygiene formed part of that curriculum. In 1929 Edith Haydon wrote in the *American Journal of Nursing* about the different ways that "mental nursing" was taught at her school at St Elizabeths. As explanation for the inclusion of mental hygiene concepts in the course, Haydon wrote that the goal of the course was "that the nurse may go out into her life's work prepared to remove prejudices existent in the public mind towards the mentally ill and towards mental institutions, and to carry forward the gospel of mental hygiene."[1] Here mental hygiene seemed to offer the profession of nursing multiple benefits, not just to improve the public image of the mental hospital but to broaden the scope of nursing practice beyond those very walls. In the most obvious sense, this conceptualization of mental hygiene resonated with the existing logic and practice of public health nursing.

Mental hygiene promised an expanded work role and a new social function that drew on nursing's own long and proud tradition. As Christine Beebe noted in the *American Journal of Nursing* in 1922, "Public health and mental hygiene go hand in hand."[2] Through mental hygiene work conceptualized as public health practice, nurses would be expanding on their options for career pathways. Importantly, Beebe pointed out that the focus in "the mental hygiene magazines" was on the role of the social worker in this space, and she argued that if nurses did not move quickly, they would find themselves shut out of this rapidly expanding area.[3] Public health was considered the natural domain of the nurse, yet the lack of education and training in mental health knowledge meant that the profession was not prepared to take up mental hygiene work. This lack of knowledge was both cause and effect of psychiatric nursing being "the most neglected arm of the profession"[4] and laid the field open to other technicians like attendants, who were mostly male, and the emerging psychiatric social workers, who threatened to take over the access to families and communities that nurses had fought so hard for.[5]

Nurses' engagement with mental hygiene was more than utilitarian, however. While mental hygiene had originated from a critique of the asylum, after World War I it was taken up by the "new psychiatrists" who saw a role for themselves in the creation of a healthy society outside the asylum walls. In their dynamic approach these psychiatrists drew on concepts from Freudian psychoanalysis and a blend of physiological and environmental theories to argue that mental health and illness were the products of environment and occurred along a spectrum from "normal" to "abnormal."[6] This conceptualization meant that mental illness was potentially everywhere, and possibly curable. For psychiatrists, this shift in focus was an overt attempt to legitimize their claims to medical authority and to dissociate themselves from the increasing criticism of custodial institutions.[7] For nurses, this promise of prevention was central to an expanded idea of nursing care in mental health that stood in sharp contrast to the work undertaken in psychiatric hospitals. One of the barriers to attracting young nurses to work in those institutions had been distaste for the nature of the work—the emphasis on custody, restraint, and the threat of violence. Generally speaking, nurses were nurses because they wanted to help people, but some expressed pessimism about the purpose of nursing work in institutions, feeling that their contribution made little difference to the prospect of cure or recovery. As caring work, institutional nursing was at times considered depressing, tiring, and even hopeless.[8] Mental hygiene work that promised the possibility of a cure and that could be exercised by the nurse herself in the everyday discharge of her duties more clearly spoke to the aspirations of a profession beginning to see itself as holding special significance for patient outcomes in mental health.

The nurse who was trained in mental hygiene concepts, it was argued, was better prepared to observe the early onset of symptoms and to recognize environments that "bred" mental health problems. She could be the ears and the eyes of the psychiatrist who rarely saw the patient outside the hospital or, increasingly, the private clinic. Nurses therefore could and would go where the psychiatrist did not. This activity would serve an important health function, potentially keeping the individual out of unpleasant hospitals and forestalling the need for acute care, and at the same time relieving the ever-increasing institutional burden. As May Kennedy argued, "Large numbers of patients could be prevented from ever getting into hospitals for the insane if our nurses had more knowledge of mental hygiene, and were prepared to give intelligent advice, at the onset of disease."[9] At the same time, mental hygiene was considered essential to the safe return of a patient to their family and community. The nurse trained in mental hygiene concepts would be a vital component of aftercare, helping the readjustment and integration of the former patient back into their regular life, and helping to monitor symptoms of a potential relapse. Mental health work conceptualized as hygiene also facilitated a discourse of "self-help" for the outpatient, who could be taught tools and skills of self-efficacy and emotional self-control on discharge from a facility.[10]

Mental hygiene as public health preventative work, with a focus on families and communities, expanded not only the places of work for nurses but the purpose of the work itself. The ability of the nurse schooled in mental hygiene to see environmental and family problems as potential mental health issues would, it was argued, serve an important community and social function. The early identification of mental health issues within a family, especially those caused by financial stress so endemic to the Great Depression, would help to alleviate potential escalations to domestic violence or self-harm. In this sense, nurses saw themselves as fulfilling not just health but social functions, referring people to services, protecting women and children, and addressing social problems. This was particularly important in the interwar years, with growing concerns about alcoholism, violence, and unemployment. Nurses made a direct connection between these circumstances and their impact on mental health, arguing that if better information and tools were available to people about how to handle their stressors and anger then much suffering could be avoided.

In a passionate and powerful article about increasing rates of depression and suicide, for example, Louise Yale lay the blame at the feet of social and medical indifference to the suffering of the mentally ill and the mistaken belief that those with illness were somehow to blame. In 1934 she argued that the mentally ill were in fact less to blame for their situation than those with typhoid fever, given "its disgusting origin," and she lamented the mentality that had made attention to mental health so little a part of nursing practice. "It is a very disturbing fact," she argued, "that so many nurses, keen enough to detect and report obscure physical symptoms of serious import, show neither recognition of nor concern regarding the simplest of depressive symptoms."[11] Nurses' own attitudes were created in and reinforced by a society and culture that held mental illness to be a sign of personal weakness. Indeed, mental illness was surrounded by a fear that was often not far removed from medieval hysteria. This shame and stigma did everyone a disservice, and was particularly galling in the nursing profession, which was so well placed to help, and be trusted by, families. It was the responsibility of nurses to know what to look for, to do and say something about what they saw, and encourage people to get help. Yale urged "nurses to disabuse themselves of the narrow and prejudiced idea that psychiatric care places a stigma upon a patient," an idea which "should have been abandoned long ago by every intelligent person, especially by educated nurses."[12]

There was no need for stigma and shame in modern conceptions of mental health and illness. Mental hygienists argued that mental health—both the normal and abnormal—existed on a continuum, that there were gradations of human behavior, that anyone could step over the line at any moment. As Haydon wrote in 1928, "The symptoms in mental disease are but exaggerations of mechanisms present in the normal individual."[13] Thus, if nurses could normalize mental health as a topic of conversation in their home visits, then they could raise awareness of symptoms and triggers, and include mental health as a regular part of health assessments and health teaching. Stigma kept mental illness in the dark, exploding through families and shattering lives, which early detection and treatment could have avoided.

The emphasis on prevention and the alleged importance of environment in mental illness also resonated with the public health nurses' focus on mothers and babies, and the emerging child guidance movement. As Gerald N. Grob has argued, "Prevention was an attractive option, particularly since it emphasized the problems related to childhood. Severely and chronically mentally ill persons often aroused hostility and rejection, whereas children—even those engaging in disruptive behavior—were perceived with compassion and sympathy."[14] To include the mental aspects of child health should have been an easy extension of nursing work. At the very least, nurses' existing role as primary care givers for mothers and children made mental hygiene a natural addition to the visiting nurse's tool kit. This was especially the case in high density urban areas where nurses were highly visible in local communities and already well established in clinics and experimenting with new demonstration projects.[15] Community services for child and family mental hygiene were largely focused on the prevention of a state of affairs commonly called "juvenile delinquency"; that is, the apparently antisocial behavior of young people leading to a life of depravity and criminality. The near obsession with delinquency in the interwar years led to the growth of the child guidance movement and the establishment of the Bureau of Child Guidance in 1922. As Dennis Doyle explains, child guidance "was an offshoot of mental hygiene. Between the 1920s and 1940s its experts helped psychologize child-rearing. Initially they were concerned with identifying and treating the emotional problems that caused juvenile delinquency. In practice child guidance was administered by an interdisciplinary team of psychiatrists, psychologists, and a new kind of mental health professional: the psychiatric social worker."[16] Notably, Doyle does not mention nurses in this scenario, and this absence was keenly felt by nurses themselves, who began to agitate for their own unique role in this interdisciplinary team.

The formal child guidance movement was still in its infancy in the 1920s but developed rapidly with money from the Commonwealth Fund and the National Committee for Mental Hygiene. By 1944 sixty clinics had been established across the country.[17] They were typically associated with the courts and aimed at addressing "delinquency" and other problem behaviors, but nurses argued that if they were trained in mental hygiene concepts then they could use their role as public health, school, and visiting nurses to prevent many of the so-called bad habits that led to this behavior. Effie Taylor maintained that "this early period of life . . . is the best time possible to establish through desirable habits and eliminate through suggestion or substitution undesirable or disadvantageous tendencies" and stressed this time was characterized by the "greatest plasticity in the human mind."[18] Nurses like V. M. Macdonald quoted from one of the founders of the child guidance movement, William Healey, in arguing for the active and positive influence of the nurse as a trusted person, not just by the parents, but children themselves, who could turn to the nurse as a confidant when things at home were problematic.[19] This was especially true for the adolescent who needed objective and scientifically based advice when it came to matters of sexuality, rather than the obfuscation of the embarrassed parent.[20] The link between sexuality and delinquency was an integral part of both mental hygiene and psychiatry in the interwar years, drawing not just on Freud but also on broader social fears about deviance and the moral fabric of American society.[21] This "child-saving" hysteria took a particular form for nurses, who saw themselves largely as "health teachers" rather than therapists. Up until the 1940s, they tried to position themselves as a trusted source of information for ignorant parents, an exemplar of good habits, and a part of the preventative project by identifying early symptoms of mental illness. Thus, they used mental hygiene concepts to argue for an expansion of their scope of practice beyond the specialist institution, but still bounded by the authority of the clinic.

The Idea of the Clinic: Harriet Bailey's *Nursing Mental Diseases*

During the early part of the twentieth century, the idea of the clinic began to take on new forms. As psychiatrists shifted their focus to prevention and private practice with middle-class "neurotics," new types of institutions such as the "psychopathic clinic" emerged. These were usually offshoots of larger institutions, often connected to those systems as training and research centers, but mostly used as small, acute-care private inpatient facilities. Two of the most famous were the Boston Psychopathic Hospital in Massachusetts (opened in 1912) and the Henry Phipps Clinic at Johns Hopkins Hospital in Baltimore (opened in 1913).[22] The first director of the Phipps Clinic was Adolf Meyer, a key figure in American psychiatry for many decades.[23] Effie Taylor was appointed as director of the Nursing Service, and Harriet Bailey as her assistant. Esther Richards, a young associate in psychiatry at Hopkins, worked closely with Taylor and Bailey to develop a curriculum, gave lectures to the student nurses, and wrote extensively about the role of the nurse. Richards recognized the importance of mental health concepts for public health and child guidance nursing, arguing that "perhaps in no field of the profession does this training in a larger conception of human needs and possibilities reap a better harvest than in the sphere of public health work" and that "the public health nurse, also, in her various associations with the child welfare movement is admirably fitted to convey the message of preventive psychiatry *if equipped with a training productive of such a point of view.*"[24] Richards was trying to make the point that psychiatric training had benefits for nursing across the spectrum of practice settings, including a better understanding of the patient as a whole. She was also a strong advocate of nurses learning more about the science of mental illness, such as it was, so that they could learn to tell the differences and connections between mental and physical distress in all nursing settings.[25] At the nurse training school at the Phipps Clinic theoretical lectures were given by Richards and then supplemented by smaller classes and clinical demonstrations.[26]

It was from this model that the first mental health text written entirely by a nurse was developed. This text was *Nursing Mental Diseases* by Harriet Bailey.[27] The timeline of Bailey's work life is unclear, however she described herself as "formerly Assistant Superintendent of Nurses at the Johns Hopkins Hospital Training School for Nurses (Henry Phipps Psychiatric Clinic) and Formerly Superintendent of Nurses, Manhattan State Hospital NY." She was a special appointment to the League of Red Cross Societies in Geneva when *Nursing Mental Diseases* appeared in 1920. Her work in that appointment focused mainly on public health,[28] but the link between public health and her approach to mental health is clearly explicated in the text. Given that this was the only such text written wholly by a nurse until 1946, and that it was frequently referenced and reviewed by other nurses, it is worth exploring in some detail.

Bailey prefaces her book with an explanation of its origins, as a "response to many requests that the writer put into more available form the subject matter of her classes with nurses."[29] The first half of the text sets out the basic concepts that informed Bailey's approach to her teaching of mental illness, and the second half details nursing procedures for various conditions. Bailey's text engages with a multitude of ideas, and she includes chapters on the causes, classifications, and symptomology of mental illnesses that are at the same time biological and environmental in focus. But it is in the chapter on prevention, and in the ways she conceptualizes the connection between biology and behavior, that we see Bailey's particular conception of the role of the nurse in mental hygiene, which she saw as an inherently social one. In the chapter on prevention she makes her case clear: "In no branch of medicine are preventive measures more insistently needed than in that of mental diseases, where the crippling of unnumbered minds with the resultant loss to society, waste in industry, expenditure of vast sums of money for care and treatment, and the weakening of the race by the transmission of infectious nervous systems, make this a social problem of exceeding importance."[30]

Leaving aside the idea of "infectious nervous systems" for the moment, this statement indicated broad thinking and an ambitious project of work for nursing. Bailey argued here, and in an article published in 1922, that through an integration of mental hygiene concepts into the general nursing curriculum nurses everywhere could learn to recognize symptoms in the hospital setting, alert the physician before a patient was dismissed, and therefore signal high-risk patients for follow-up or referral to other services.[31] This was also the case for public health nurses, because, Bailey argued, "it is known that much of mental illness could be averted or checked if prophylaxis had begun in early years, or been applied when symptoms first appeared."[32] The public health nurse with mental hygiene training could be "one of the most important and forceful agents in this field" because she had access to people at all stages of life, including those without any signs of mental illness. She could inquire into their home, family, and work life noting potential hazards, stressors, and "bad habits," and she was able to "call attention to these matters without giving offence."[33]

This level of concern with the everyday life of the family existed in the context of a whole-society surveillance of the moral character of American communities. Bailey made overt references to prohibition, new drug laws, and concerns with "sex delinquency" to argue for mental health based on "a practise [sic] of the single standard of morality—a pure life for men as well as for women."[34] In her role as a trusted adviser then, the nurse could help the family make "improvements in hygienic conditions," including suggestions about food, clothing, exercise, environment, and interpersonal conflicts. This last was particularly important—through the observation of family dynamics the nurse trained in mental hygiene "may be able to make suggestions for readjustments which will relieve the stress and strain and promote the health and happiness of the whole household."[35] In this sense, Bailey was a strong advocate of child guidance work. The nurse who was trusted by a family, and by extension a local community, could intervene in "parental difficulties and conflicts" with advice and suggestions. For Bailey, good parenting involved striking a balance between "coddling" and adequately protecting a child from experiences that could form trauma. At the same time, the child should be fully socialized in order to learn the principles of healthy relationships: "truthfulness, honesty, unselfishness, generosity, patience, gentleness and courtesy."[36] With consistent, loving, and firm parenting, the "plastic mind" of the child could be made resilient and adaptable, and build a character of self-control and self-reliance. Bailey stressed the importance of childhood for future mental health, arguing that "children and youths whose mental strength has thus been conserved and cultivated will more easily meet and efficiently overcome the difficulties presented by the changes and readjustments which inevitably are a part of every life."[37] The focus on concepts such as plasticity and resilience reflected the idea that human beings needed to adapt to rapidly changing social circumstances, particularly ways of working.

The demanding nature of new industrial forms of work informed by "scientific management" techniques like Taylorism and Fordism were of interest to many social science and psychological experts in the interwar years. Scientific management's promise of efficiency and progress was seen as central to the rebuilding of American democracy and prosperity, but they required a certain kind of worker, someone who could adapt to the discipline of the clock and the production line, and this required a stable mind and sound personal habits.[38] In phrases prescient of Freud's still-to-be-published *Civilization and Its Discontents*, Bailey maintained that work could be a source of both sublimation of the instincts and rewards both material and intellectual. "The daily performance of some appointed task or duty which engages the time and the attention is one of the most valuable means for the preservation and promotion of mental health,"[39] she argued. The stress of modern work needed to be balanced with recreation, rest, and creativity, but it was also important that the type of work be suited to the personality. An industrial nurse trained in mental hygiene could spot early warning signs of "the effects of uncongenial work . . . for feelings of bitterness, antagonism and rebellion are often created which tend to warp the ideas, crush initiative and ambition and paralyze energy and activity."[40]

An emphasis on the character building nature of work also informed Bailey's advice for nurses working in mental hospitals, and stemmed from Meyer's great belief in "occupational therapy."[41] While he did not invent the term or the practice, he is often credited with its rise to prominence in the United States,[42] but in reality work had a long history in psychiatry. It had been one of the therapeutic tenets of "moral treatment" dating back to the 1700s and had been in use at the Quaker asylums in the United States since the early 1800s.[43] But it was Meyer who most influenced Bailey's work: in the second section of her text, which focuses on the actual nursing practices related to the care of the mentally ill in institutions, Meyer's concept of occupational therapy features prominently. In each of the chapters that deal with the technical aspects of nursing for the various types of illness, a section is dedicated to "Occupation," which covers any kind of activity that uses the patient's mind or hands. Activities might range from music, singing, reading, knitting, weaving, painting, card games, and bowling to dancing, gymnastics, and outdoor yardwork for the men. The aim with this kind of work was not simply to divert or entertain the patient, but, with careful encouragement, to rebuild the person's damaged sense of self and return the person to some kind of functional reality. Bailey points out that the interested sympathy of the nurse is central because no two patients will respond to the same activity, and the nurse must use her skills of getting to know the patient to find an activity that is suited to them and not triggering of past failure or trauma. At the same time, these activities were designed to rebuild the healthy habit neural pathways, and needed to be performed with kindness and patience from the nurse. This understanding of the context and life history of the patient was central to Bailey's conceptualization of mental hygiene.

Despite the destigmatizing and empathic elements of Bailey's work on mental hygiene, there are tensions between the theoretical ideal and the practical reality. As Grob has argued, "Based on the belief that it was possible and easier to prevent mental disorders than it was to cure them . . . mental hygiene was an attractive concept . . . consistent with the effort to expand the role and authority of psychiatry in American life."[44] And while it attempted to draw on new scientific knowledge to do so, it was still the case that mental hygiene "was but a continuation of a venerable religious tradition that stressed natural law, free will, and individual responsibility."[45] This belief in prevention, and the work that surrounded it, also signaled a tension between psychiatrists and the continued existence of the mental hospital, from which the profession was growing increasingly distant. It was obvious to many that "the intractable problems of the severely and chronically mentally ill"[46] would not be solved by psychiatry as it currently existed, and that mental hygiene itself had little to offer this type of patient. Mental hygiene was not practical or useful within the confines of the large hospital where most of the actual care took place, thus whatever the role mental hygiene could have played in nursing, there was neither capacity nor the infrastructure with which to implement it. More than this, however, was a tension inherent to the very concept of mental hygiene, which appeared to be empathetic, destigmatizing, and nonjudgmental but was in fact dangerously close to being otherwise. When Bailey referred to "infectious nervous systems" she was alluding to a distinct thread within mental hygiene that stressed not just environment but heredity.

The stretch from mental hygiene to eugenics was not a long one, in fact Meyer himself had been on the advisory council of the American Eugenics Society from 1912 to 1935.[47] While Meyer may not have supported the link between psychiatry and immigration restriction,[48] Bailey herself made clear reference to involuntary sterilization of the mentally ill. In the middle of her otherwise sympathetic chapter on "The Prevention of Mental Illness," Bailey includes the following paragraph:

In the prevention of mental deficiency, segregation is recognized as a most important measure for these individuals have not the mental qualities which make them valuable to society, and economically they are a partial or total loss, but especially because it is an established fact that this type of defective family increases at about double the rate of the general population, and feeblemindedness is inherited, for parents cannot transmit to their children nervous and mental strength which is not theirs to give. Some states have already enacted laws which provide for the sterilization of the socially unfit—the criminal, the feebleminded and the incurably insane.[49]

Later in the text Bailey adds to this comment by drawing on current social thinking that was almost obsessive about the link between delinquency, criminality, and mental illness. As was so evident in the child guidance movement, the belief that delinquency (unproblematically defined) was hereditary (as opposed to normal youthful exuberance or a logical effect of social circumstances) led to some dangerous thinking about ways in which to treat not just the mentally ill but the "mentally deficient."[50] This catchall phrase included anyone who sat outside rigid norms of social functioning or productivity, as well as those with anything from mild developmental disabilities (idiocy or feeblemindedness) to the physically deformed "cretin."

In a twist that reveals the theoretical weakness at the heart of mental hygiene, Bailey writes that "the control and prevention of mental deficiency is one of the great problems of mental hygiene, for statistics show that tramps, criminals, wayward girls, paupers and the very large dependent class are to a more or less degree mentally deficient."[51] Rather than address the social circumstances that caused the mentally ill to be homeless, or critique the labels that classified the merely poor as "defective," Bailey drew on research like that of eugenicist Henry Goddard and his 1912 study of the Kallikak family, which claimed "irrefutable proof . . . that of all classes of defectives those with mental enfeeblement must surely transmit the defect."[52] In a frightening harbinger of the extreme rhetoric that would form the Nazi justification for mass murder of the developmentally disabled, Bailey wrote, "This group of unfortunates must be segregated if the problem is ever to be solved."[53] The troubling tensions in this conception of mental hygiene are hidden behind seemingly neutral scientific language, which was central to establishing the legitimacy of psychiatry as a social project.

In attempting to eradicate the last vestiges of quackery from the perception of psychiatry while at the same time validating its role as a social intervention,

psychiatrists tried to balance the objectivity of science with a continued moral-
izing about environment. It is not the case that new scientific understandings
suddenly replaced moralistic judgments or the emphasis on behavior and environment. In fact, this period saw a solidification of the connection between the
mental and physical at many levels—structurally, biologically, and socially.[54]
Bailey's text again is instructive in how these elements were conceptualized as
coexisting and as affecting each other, and her book went into some detail in an
attempt to have nurses understand the link between the brain and behavior. Her
aim was twofold: to have nurses understand that science, rather than "badness,"
was at the root of individual behavior, and that nursing actions needed to be
related to that science in order to bring about the required outcomes.

The theoretical underpinnings of Bailey's text demonstrated the way that
scientific understandings of the brain combined with Freudian influenced theories of behavior and environment. In her first chapter, called "Psychological
Introduction," Bailey lay the foundation for mental health within the "nervous
system," in which memory, thought, feeling, and action are laid down in neural
pathways through repetition, what she called "association paths" in which "each
repetition tends to make the pathway more deep and lasting."[55] However, there
is a tension between what the conscious mind and the unconscious mind pay
attention to, and therefore habits are sometimes reflexive rather than deliberate
choices. As she noted, "Psychologists have estimated that not more than one in
ten of our waking acts is the result of conscious choice or volition."[56] The need
for a repression of the instincts caused by environmental and social factors that
require the person to adjust or adapt was considered the main driving force in
this mental process, and the degree to which a person could make these necessary adjustments was the degree to which they would thrive or flounder.

Although her explanation of psychological processes sounded decidedly
Freudian, Bailey did not reference him. Her main references for this psychological approach came from William James's *Psychology: The Briefer Course*, a
highly influential text at the time. These concepts coexisted with a more neuro-
logical approach in which the brain was conceived as plastic and alterable
through intervention and readjustment. In this conceptualization, Bailey was
again most heavily influenced by Meyer, as both a theorist and clinician. Meyer
was the exemplar and leader of what Grob has called "a new psychiatry."[57]
While he drew on both Freud and Emil Kraepelin, Meyer increasingly moved
away from a classic psychoanalytic approach and rejected what he saw as dogma
for a particularly American brand of psychiatry personified by its pragmatism.
In 1917 Meyer had written that "our new world environment has been too readily overawed by the formulations of Kraepelin, Freud and others, much to the

detriment of the fresh and courageous pragmatism which is the sanest product of our best leaders."[58] This "pragmatism" was really an eclectic mix of nomenclature, science (such as it was), psychoanalysis, and related experimental treatments that together formed Meyer's psychobiological approach. This was an approach that "rejected any kind of dualism between the mind and body."[59] According to Grob, by "stressing the interaction of organism and environment, [Meyer] defined mental disorders in behavioral terms and traced their origins to defective habits."[60] Thus the science in Bailey's book placed mental processes firmly in the brain, but always reinforced by the significance of environment and the ability of the brain to change, adapt, and be "retrained."

Bailey sought to explain some of the etiology of mental illness and therefore to educate her readers about which illnesses were likely to be receptive to therapeutic intervention and potential prevention. Chapter 4 of Bailey's text is entitled "Causes—General Classification of Mental Diseases," and in it she argued that understanding the causes of mental illness was central to modern psychiatric practice and its attempt to move beyond "a fund of tradition, superstition, and prejudice which unfortunately has persisted in various forms almost to the present moment."[61] Bailey argued that "advances made through medical research and the scientific study of mental disorders have enabled the psychiatrist to know definitely the direct, specific, and unmistakable causes of certain types or groups of mental disease, to know also the course which they are likely to take, in how far they will yield to treatment, and the means to which they may be prevented."[62] In reality, there was no such consensus within psychiatry about the "definite" nature of existing knowledge; in fact, many, like Meyer, actively "resisted efforts at definitive conclusions."[63] Bailey provided no references for her own classification, which uses four groupings: Organic, Toxic, Somatic Disease, and Constitutional.[64] In this classification we see some of the tensions inherent to Bailey's thinking, and the limits of psychiatric knowledge at the time. If nurses were supposed to appreciate that mental illness was a biological dysfunction like any other in an attempt to destigmatize both the patient and the mental health professions, Bailey's classification nevertheless shows an inherent emphasis on mental illnesses that were behavioral, and therefore changeable in some way.

The dubious distinctions between Bailey's four groupings meant that some illnesses were seen as more treatable than others, or more amenable to environmental or individual interventions, especially around habit formation. In the organic, toxic and infectious-exhaustive disorders, Bailey described nursing procedures that are mostly related to general nursing—feeding, bathing, temperature control, but performed with awareness of possible emotional triggers. In these sections she focuses on the use of occupational therapy as diversion, and the role of the nurse is limited to these kind ministrations.

It is in the constitutional psychoses classification that we see the blend of science and environment, and the intermingling of mental hygiene concepts with new approaches. By beginning this section with "A well-known physician has said: 'A cheerful, intelligent nurse of good judgment can do more for these patients than all the doctors and drugs in creation,'" Bailey emphasized the therapeutic power of the nurse herself.[65] The nurse's attitude with the patient was paramount—Bailey stressed the singular role of the nurse as a gentle but firm "mother substitute" (while warning against excessive coddling and the possibility of transference). Kindness and patience were vital—the nurse working with depressed, melancholic, manic, or schizophrenic patients must put aside her own frustrations and beliefs and be aware of how her own demeanor can either reinforce negative behaviors and paranoias or build new experiences through a trusting relationship. But there was more to the nursing procedures here than basic care. It was through conversations with patients that the nurse could challenge old ideas and replace them with new habits, laying down new neural pathways and associations. "Re-education," she argued, "includes all the measures which are taken to develop the latent capacities and to correct old and erroneous new habits."[66] Apart from kindness, patience, and occupational therapy, however, what was the nurse specifically meant to *do* in this re-education process?

Bailey did not see an autonomous therapeutic role for the nurse. While her everyday nursing actions, as well as her personality and interactions with the patient, should in and of themselves be constructive and rehabilitative rather than reinforcing of past trauma, the nurse's therapeutic capacities were limited to conversation, diversion, and occupation. This did not mean that she should be ignorant of other therapeutic treatments, however. It was simply that the nurse herself would not apply them. Rather, she needed to know how psychotherapy or psychoanalysis was being used by the physician, because her job was to supplement "his efforts . . . so that she may more intelligently carry out the special orders, make more accurate observations, secure fuller cooperation and thereby insure better results from the patient. A physicians efforts may be nullified by a nurse who does not know or understand the principles of treatment."[67]

In the same way, Bailey continued to justify the use of both hydrotherapy and restraint, although the use of restraint, she noted, was on the decline, with some hospitals forbidding its use outright. Again, it was a treatment at the level of the physician, and the nurse's job was to ensure the patients comfort and safety: "Only in extreme cases of excitement, when no appeal is comprehended, and the patient becomes a danger to himself and other patients, the physician orders the application of the protection or safety sheet. . . . During this treatment the patient must be watched carefully."[68] The following chapter was then devoted to the application of hydrotherapy as a nursing procedure, because "water has long been valued as a nerve stimulant, sedative, and general tonic."[69] In many ways, Bailey merely reflected the reality of working with limited tools at this time. There was no framework yet by which nurses could position themselves as therapists, nor would there have been social acceptance for such an idea. It was as yet barely thinkable that a nurse might question the physician's judgment or approach, and in many ways Bailey's work signaled the desire and aspirations of nurses who would like to do more in mental health work but who had neither the knowledge nor the power to do so.

Bailey's text therefore was aimed at changing what she could but is still very much a product of its time. It nevertheless stood unchallenged for twenty years in terms of texts written by and for nurses. The main goal of the book, and of her work more broadly, was summed up in the long paragraph that concludes the chapter on "Psychological Introduction," explaining why an understanding of the science of mental illness, such as it was at the time, was considered so important for nurses everywhere:

It is hoped that the student nurse will have learned something about the laws which control human thought and conduct, and realize that for everything in the mental life, every thought, every feeling, every action, there is a reason, which will make her more tolerant of and sympathetic with peculiarities in the behavior of patients under her care who otherwise would appear uninteresting, unreasonable and disagreeable; that she will be more eager to understand the causes of abnormal mental activity, and to have a part in the restoration to health of those who are mentally ill, for to her is afforded the extraordinary opportunity of supplementing the physician's efforts to modify and change tendencies and characteristics which may be harmful, to hold ever before the patient the ideals and conduct as will help him attain them, and so secure for him the greatest measure of health, happiness, usefulness and efficiency in the future.[70]

In this paragraph, Bailey articulates the ideal type of psychiatric nurse, a characterization that stood in opposition to what actually existed, and also demonstrates the strong disciplining and normalizing tendencies in psychiatric thinking at this point in history.

Toward Holistic Nursing

While Bailey was writing specifically for nurses attending training schools within psychiatric hospitals or short courses attached to regular nursing programs, the significance of mental health concepts went beyond the asylum walls. For many nursing leaders, mental hygiene was not simply synonymous with what would come to be called "community mental health"; rather, it was an aspect of nursing care in all settings. As Frances Thielbar argued, "We wish our students to carry their knowledge of mental hygiene and mental nursing into the whole nursing field and apply the principle of caring for the whole individual in the general hospital and in the public health field."[71] Bailey had stressed this idea of treating the "whole individual" because "physical and mental disorders cannot always be separated by sharp lines of demarcation."[72] This meant that mental health concepts were important for all nursing.

These were ideas that Effie Taylor advocated in her writing and leadership through the early part of the twentieth century as director of nursing at Phipps, then as faculty and dean of nursing at Yale as well as president of both the National League for Nursing Education (NLNE) and the International Council of Nurses. Mental hygiene was central to her thinking, but it was a much more expansive conceptualization than simply prevention. In 1926 she argued "it is imperative that all nurses have an understanding of the patient as a whole and there is no such thing as mental nursing apart from general nursing or general nursing apart from mental nursing. They form a oneness and make up the whole."[73] For Taylor, this was a scientific reality: "From our knowledge of how the whole organism acts, it is obvious that what affects one part affects the other and a sense of well-being or ill being in either the mind or the body brings about reactions which are not confined to one part alone but affect the whole human being."[74] Therefore, it was imperative that nurses understood not just the signs and symptoms of mental illness or the mental or emotional aspects of physical illness, but also how they were in fact intimately connected. At the most basic level, this understanding was essential for all nurses because it facilitated "an understanding of the mental factors entering into the human adjustment and is equally as necessary to use in caring for patients in the general hospital as in the special hospital."[75] If mental nursing and general nursing were to be linked to each other in this way, it was because physical and mental health themselves could not be separated, and neither could they be separated from the social and environmental context in which they occurred. For nurses writing in the 1920s through the 1940s, this conception of mental illness had ramifications for patient care, for the profession, and for society more broadly.

In their insistence on the significance of mental health concepts, nurses often focused on patient care and outcomes within general hospitals and not just psychiatric ones. As early as 1922, for example, nurses like Christine Beebe argued that "the nurse meets the mental and nervous element in every case of physical disease or injury with which she comes into contact, but never having been taught to recognize this element, its significance escapes her."[76] She lamented that this lack of knowledge had "wrought actual injury to many nervous cases that we encountered in medical or surgical work," and, at the same time, lack of knowledge about psychiatric concepts meant that "we failed entirely to get the right point of view" when dealing with psychologically distressed patients in either the general or mental hospital setting.[77] In the same vein, May Kennedy wrote that "if nurses in the general hospital had even a few months' training in psychiatry they would be able to treat all abnormal cases with greater intelligence and much mental misery of the patient might be avoided."[78] While Kennedy here may be talking about the ability to pinpoint potential cases of escalating mental illness, other nurses lamented the damage that had been and continued to be done by nurses not recognizing that a patient's behavior in general hospital may be because of psychological issues either underlying or as an effect of physical conditions.

Katherine McLean argued that not understanding the perfectly normal psychological aspects of physical illness could also lead to dire consequences: "If you have a patient who, after many physical illnesses, is unable to rise above his symptoms and pain, how easy it is to stamp him as neurotic and to spoil hope of recovery for him."[79] The inability to recognize what was too often called problem behavior as either an effect of physical distress or as a sign of impending mental illness meant that patients were dismissed as "difficult" and not treated properly, causing a spiral effect. Some nurses argued that psychiatric training meant that nurses would be better positioned to observe when a patient was suffering prolonged or "abnormal" distress in relation to physical illness that may require psychiatric intervention, while others argued that nurses simply needed to understand that all physical illnesses had a psychological aspect. Tina Duerksen, for example, insisted that "one of the major needs and problems in nursing today is a better understanding of human nature especially during illness, the recognition that the mental and physical aspects of disease are inseparable."[80] This awareness of the connection between the mental and physical was essential for whole patient care.

Kennedy, who was active as both a consultant to the American Psychiatric Association and chairperson of the NLNE's psychiatric nursing committees,[81] made this connection explicit when she asked, "When is nursing 'mental nursing?' It is true that there are patients who are suffering from disturbances which are pronounced deviations from normal mental well-being, but then I would like to drop the term 'mental nursing' and say 'nursing the patient.' We do not say 'physical nursing.' All sick people are mentally and physically impaired and they all need the care of a nurse who understands both aspects of their illness."[82] For nurse leaders like Kennedy and Taylor, the fact that this was *not* the standard reality of nursing practice was a cause of great concern.

For Taylor especially, the fact that the nurse (psychiatric or otherwise) was not already practicing in a holistic way was a source of embarrassment and frustration. She was less concerned with whether social workers or public health professionals were encroaching on traditional nursing space and more concerned with what was essential for a mature profession. In articulating what her Hopkins colleague Esther Richards had called "the nurse of tomorrow,"[83] Taylor wrote, "I do not think the vital question to determine is whether nurses or social workers should be responsible"[84] for advancing psychiatric practice beyond the hospital and into the community but whether nurses themselves were prepared for the work. Taylor did not think they were, and not entirely through their own fault. "The deficiency," she noted, "is not necessarily in the nurse herself, the deficiency is more obviously in her preparation which is the direct result of the system upon which nursing education in the average school is practiced, and the system is based on an immediate need, specific relations, and past traditions."[85] This lack of forethought and immaturity in the preparation of nurses meant that, as Taylor saw it, the nurse "is not adequately prepared to function intelligently in situations demanding more than that required of a skilled technician."[86] While she felt this was true of all nursing, it was especially true for nurses hoping to work meaningfully in mental health, because it was dangerous for the profession, for patients, and for the nurse herself. "It is inconceivable," Taylor argued, "that she should be debarred from gaining the knowledge which alone will prepare her to adequately function in her field."[87]

It was not just that psychiatric concepts were essential for patient care; they were also required for the mature flourishing of the nurse herself, both in mental health and beyond. For psychiatric nursing in particular, leaders like Bailey, Kennedy, and Taylor stressed the importance of maturity and self-awareness in the nurse for successful practice. Importantly, they argued, mental health care was not just something that happened to and for other people but an essential part of actually being a psychiatric nurse. How could the nurse adequately help others to deal with emotional distress, to recover, to grow, mature, and flourish if she was not in control of her own emotional state? This maturity was necessary in order to move psychiatric nursing beyond its traditional custodial function, and was essential for the destigmatizing of both mental patients and the mental health professions. As such, nurse leaders argued that there was no moral or individual choice element to mental illness, and nursing needed to let go of the old attitudes that hampered patient care: "Like most people who know nothing about psychoses, we covered our dread of this thing with a laugh and looked upon these patients not as sick but as absurdities to be hidden away behind walls and forgotten about as much as possible."[88] This type of behavior on behalf of the nurse did the profession as a whole a disservice, and indicated a lack of maturity in the nurse, whose job it was to put her own feelings aside and provide the best care possible.

Knowledge about mental illness was essential to this process. As Bailey argued, "When one understands even imperfectly the mechanisms which govern behavior and speech and sees the manifestations of disordered mechanism, one surely tends to become more charitable, more patient, more sympathetic with the patients who are difficult, peculiar or 'queer' and whose symptoms have proved annoying, exasperating and vexing."[89] The frequency with which nurse leaders spoke to the significance of psychiatric knowledge for dealing with judgmentalism and stigma can be taken as an indication of the frequency with which this kind of behavior occurred. Nurses were not making a case for psychiatric education because nurses were already working well in this space, but because in fact they were not. Rather, the profession was marred, and patient care substandard, because of the judgments that nurses themselves brought to psychiatric work. At the very least it was hoped that knowledge about and exposure to psychiatric patients would begin to shift preconceived ideas about the mentally ill.

It was to this end that Katherine McLean reported on the course she ran at Boston Psychopathic Hospital, in which student nurses reported feeling more optimistic and less afraid. One student wrote, "Above all else, I have learned to be patient, more tolerant, less rapid to draw conclusions or to abide by first impressions."[90] Kennedy noted that fear of mental illness was itself a barrier to attracting nurses to the profession: "It is appalling to learn how many competent, sympathetic, and conscientious nurses are registered against mental cases because they have had no training in psychiatry. They do not understand the affliction and are afraid."[91] Knowledge and experience were the keys to overcoming this fear, and, it was hoped, they would also lead to a more mature nurse all round.

Edith Haydon similarly hoped that more education and exposure in psychiatric work would mean that the nurse would develop a deeper understanding of her own emotional life and behavior.[92] She argued that with proper education "the nurse should have a more thorough understanding of her own reactions, and those of her patients and friends. She should be broader minded and more tolerant."[93] Similarly, Myra Whitney argued that even a brief course in psychiatric nursing would help the nurse "to understand her own reactions . . . [and] assist her in understanding and aiding all maladjusted individuals as well as being a benefit to herself in helping to maintain a sane and balanced attitude toward her own problems."[94] This knowledge would benefit the nurse herself and, it was hoped, flow through to her practice.

By stressing the humanity and individuality of the patient, Thielbar argued that a well-structured educational program could teach more than the technical aspects of mental health nursing and "create an attitude toward the patient" whereby it was recognized that patients were still people, that they had had full and complex lives before they became patients, and that the fact of their being in a psychiatric hospital did not make them any less of a person who should be treated with respect and dignity.[95] As Louise Yale reminded her readers, it could very well be a family member that the nurse came to treat one day, and so it was necessary that she put aside her own preconceived ideas and fears. She urged nurses to "preserve an open and intelligent attitude toward psychiatry" in order to "clear away some of the misinformation and misconceptions current among the general public, not forgetting that her own friends and relatives are part of the general public."[96]

Mental Hygiene for American Society

New concepts of psychiatry and mental health required nurses to recognize the impact of childhood experiences on emotional development and to put these experiences in their broader social context. In much of their writing through the 1920s and 1930s, nurses talked about mental illness as a problem of adjustment to social pressures and norms. They clearly recognized the particular stresses inherent to American life in the interwar period and placed the blame for increased rates of depression and suicide at the feet of the economic crises of the Great Depression.[97] They argued that psychiatric preparation meant that nurses could make meaningful contributions to the care of the individual and the family if these factors were properly recognized and understood. In their role as nurses, with more access to patients and families than any other profession, they had a unique opportunity to contribute to the science of human behavior. At the most obvious level, scientific advances in mental health required the active participation of nurses, whose notes were an important part of the diagnosis of conditions and whose assistance in the collection of data across multiple cases would help to advance knowledge more broadly.[98] As Effie

Taylor argued in her presidential address to the NLNE in 1935, the mental health nurse of tomorrow would be part of an important social and scientific project in which she would be perceived as a "scientific worker, questioning in her interest, trained to lead and to teach intelligently. She is also prepared by education to assist the physicians and research workers, who are striving through investigation, observation and study to find new knowledge through which to protect and preserve the health of our people."[99] This was a particular concern in the shadow of war, which Taylor characterized as a kind of collective psychosis. "We find the world today," she argued, "in its present chaotic state largely because we are not able to interpret the thinking of each other; we are not able to understand the effect which mental attitudes have upon our bodily reactions. . . . Conflict and strife seem uppermost . . . in world relations, and it may be because our people are fearful of themselves and each other."[100]

By "our people" Taylor did not just mean the American people, but humanity more broadly. In an earlier paper she had explicitly linked nurses' work in mental health to the worldwide project of peace and happiness. "The immediate question," she argued, "is how can nurses be prepared to do the work which is knocking at their door so loudly. . . . Over 100,000 nurses daily are making sickness and health contacts and every contact presupposes a mental as well as a physical life. These contacts include human beings of every age, race and social status. Every unobserved or unrecognized symptom is a lost opportunity to insure a healthier, happier and more efficient human race."[101] This idea of efficiency was particularly central and intimately connected to the political project of American democracy. Mental stability was necessary for social stability, and mental efficiency was essential to American productivity, at both the individual and group level. As Bailey argued, "The day is long past when mental weakness and illness can be ignored as a cause of or contributing factor to ill health, inefficiency and inability to bear one's part in the struggle for existence and the onward march of progress."[102] The instability and economic stresses of the interwar years gave way to very real fears about the fabric of American society as World War II loomed.

In the face of fascism and tyranny, psychiatric nurses had an even more important role to play in recognizing and fostering the individuality that was the strength of American society, and in the shoring up of mental reserves in preparation for the war to come. For Esther Anderson, writing at the beginning of American's involvement in World War II, this meant a commitment to service, social responsibility, and justice for the mentally ill, as she appealed to American nurses to do and be better. "It is well to remember the goal of professional nursing organizations," she argued, which were "to weave the mental hospitals into the picture of our total responsibilities to the communities we serve. We have not yet taken to bombing the habitations of the 'unfit' in our society"[103]—a direct reference to the medical programs of Nazi Germany, which included euthanasia of the disabled and mentally ill. Anderson reminded her readers that a rise in the recognition of mental illness did not mean that society was crumbling. Rather, new knowledge about psychiatric processes meant that "our civilization is provided with new insights applicable to the challenge before us to make democracy work."[104] The knowledge and practice of the psychiatric nurse meant "that we can appreciate realistically the sound values of individual freedoms and plan more effectively to protect them. Health, social security, and morale are closely linked and interrelated."[105] Mental health, therefore, was foundational to American success.

Surveillance and Control

In these writings, nurse leaders before World War II anticipated many of the threads and themes that would emerge through the cauldron of war. Not the least of these is the inherently normalizing role of the psychiatric discourses. For all their writing and thinking about compassion and individuality, all of this work presupposes the idea that there is such a thing as "normal" human behavior that is essential to the smooth functioning of American democracy and capitalism, and that nursing work in psychiatry should, where possible, have the social function of returning the patient to this state of normal from which they have deviated—that the person can and must learn to adjust and adapt. This is the most striking part of all of the nurse scholarship related to mental health in the prewar period: the assumption of a desirable normal. Despite a recognition of the biological origins of much disease, the arguments against stigma and superstition, and the concern with the patient as a whole person, psychiatric nursing in this period was still very much about surveillance and control. The role of the nurse was to advise, teach, report, and observe signs and symptoms of problems of adjustment, maladaptation, bad habits, deviant sexuality, depression—anything that might signal a threat to productivity, efficiency, and "happiness." The advice that nurses were being asked to give patients and parents was based on a culturally, socially, and politically constructed idea of an American normal that was never defined, always assumed. In many ways this was an effect of the emphasis on mental hygiene in their thinking. By nature it was an ideology and technique aimed at normalizing and controlling, even going so far as to inform eugenic thought and justifying reproductive engineering. While Bailey has been lauded by some as an influential nurse leader, this aspect of her work in particular remains hidden and problematic.[106]

While nurses recognized the potential of public health work as a form of community mental health, their primary place of work was in fact the specialist psychiatric institution, which was not even remotely on the decline in this period. The hospital remained the central and actual location of their work. That they sought to reform the conditions and the nature of the nursing work in those institutions is notable, but it is also the case that they never questioned the asylum as a place of control, and neither did they speak publicly about what we now know where in fact terrible conditions. If new nurses were afraid to join the psychiatric profession it was for good reason—overcrowding, violence, restraint, chaos, and a very real lack of recovery marked the psychiatric institution of the early twentieth century, and very few graduating nurses chose psychiatric hospitals as their place of work or home. Mental hygiene was attractive not least because it opened avenues for work outside the institution.

Nurses did become increasingly aware in this period of the need for mental health concepts across the whole spectrum of nursing practice, and of the urgent need for the development of advanced practice in psychiatry, but they were faced with the sharp reality of a lack of courses, a lack of uniformity in the courses that did exist, and structural and attitudinal barriers to the development of same. In reality, public health nurses were unprepared for mental health work because of the focus on institutional care, in both general and mental nursing. Psychiatric nursing concepts remained disconnected from general nursing training, and, as a result, the field remained open to the development of other professions like the psychiatric social worker and the occupational therapist. Bailey and Kennedy made some attempt to articulate the importance of the nurse-patient relationship but, lacking theoretical rigor, this translated in practice into occupational therapy. Most nurse scholars in this period did not make the leap to defining nursing practice as actively therapeutic because the focus in training was on the basic nursing tasks, so despite their rhetoric about the connection between mental and physical health, nurses had no real tools apart from advice to be kind and compassionate with which to actively address mental aspects of illness. The nursing scholarship in this period is important, however, because it clearly locates the problem in this very lack of knowledge and training, and recognizes the barriers and issues within the current structures of nurse education. At the same time as they wrote about what needed to change, and what the potential for psychiatric nursing could and should be, many of these nurses were actively working to create the educational structures that would make the next step possible. These developments are the subject of chapter 3.

"The Nurse of Tomorrow"

Creating Advanced Practice Courses in Psychiatry

The interwar period had revealed a number of structural and ideological obstacles to the development of psychiatric nursing as a profession. While mental hygiene may have resonated with the image of the public health nurse, it was still the case that most mental health work took place in institutions. These institutions continued to be fully controlled by psychiatrists, and the "in-house" nature of training programs for their attendant and nursing staff rankled with professional nursing associations. They were seen as substandard in that they did not provide a broad enough education for graduates to be considered registered nurses, and their physical location and conditions remained unattractive to newly qualified nurses, who were in high demand. Despite the protestations of psychiatrists, mental health institutions were highly stigmatized and feared places of work. And while mental hygiene may have seemed like a natural fit for the public health nurse, in reality mental health concepts were not included in their education.

Nurse leaders were keenly aware of the need for a revision of educational programs so that nurses could acquire the knowledge they needed to improve conditions for patients and the nursing care they received. For many of the nurses writing in the interwar period, the only satisfactory answer would be the establishment of standalone psychiatric or mental health courses embedded within university-based programs. There was, however, no real consensus on how this should happen. Many nurses argued that psychiatric nursing should be present at both the undergraduate and graduate level as it was both basic and specialist knowledge. They also argued that psychiatric nursing should be taught using curriculums established and accredited by nursing bodies themselves, but this would require the transfer of power away from psychiatrists and their training schools to nursing organizations and teachers. Before 1936 the focus was largely on integrating psychiatric concepts into the existing structures of basic nurse education (and away from hospital training schools), but the outbreak of World War II and its emphasis on the mental health of soldiers highlighted the need for specialist, advanced education for clinical psychiatric work. With the passing of the Bolton Act in 1943 (and subsequently the National Mental Health Act in 1946), the funds finally became available to address education for psychiatric work at multiple levels.

Despite this release of funds, the establishment of graduate courses in particular did not happen overnight. Many of the nurses featured in chapter 2, who had written so stridently about the need for mental health concepts to be integrated into nurse education, were also actively working to make that idea a reality. Psychiatrist Esther Richards, writing in the 1920s, had high hopes for the "nurse of tomorrow" in this regard.[1] This chapter looks beyond the published work of nurses to explore the activities of professional organizations and committees, which set the groundwork for the establishment of university-based courses. This groundwork required the negotiation of long-running sets of relationships and often competing motivations. It meant continuing to work with the American Psychiatric Association (APA) and other funding bodies like the Rockefeller Foundation while at the same time advocating for the ultimate control of nursing organizations over nursing standards and practice. In each of these relationships, nurses used growing concerns about the nation's mental health as leverage. Anxiety about the psychological condition of returned soldiers and the stressors cause by interwar social and economic instability provided the conditions for the rise of the nurse as an advanced health professional and a force of social good. Nurses were well aware of that context and knew it was central to their push for legitimacy and authority. At the same time, they were well aware of the deficiencies in both patient care and nurse education in psychiatry, and used their political and social leverage as justification for the establishment of nurse-led, university-based courses. This chapter focuses on the period from the late 1930s to the end of World War II and explores the work of committees and projects that aimed to articulate the content and structure of advanced courses for nurse education in psychiatry. In this process nurse leaders drew directly on ideas that had already been articulated in the engagement with mental hygiene and sought to find ways to operationalize those ideas into practice.

The Committee on Mental Hygiene and Psychiatric Nursing

In the previous chapters we have seen the extent to which nurses were connected to the activities and requirements of psychiatrists through the APA. Many of the nurses writing articles about the importance of mental hygiene and psychiatric concepts for nursing practice and education were at one time also members of the APA's Committee on Nursing and had well-established relationships with that organization and its members. Harriet Bailey, Effie Taylor, and May Kennedy all attended meetings of the APA and reported back from that committee to the National League for Nursing Education (NLNE) at its annual conferences. It was also the case that the nursing organizations had had their own approach to issues of mental hygiene and psychiatric work, separately of the APA. Both the NLNE and American Nurses Association (ANA) had had committees on mental hygiene since 1916—Effie Taylor was the first chair while she was also secretary of the NLNE.[2] These committees achieved little at the time partly because there was no clear consensus on what should be done or how to do it, and partly because there were no independent financial means through which to bring about any of the changes Taylor and her colleagues argued were necessary. They wrote frequently in the *American Journal of Nursing*, as we have already seen, but World War I and the subsequent Great Depression meant that American society had priorities other than the reorganization of psychiatric nursing.

At the 1933 meeting of the APA's Committee on Nursing, however, the NLNE's representative Anna McGibbon met with the committee chair, Daniel Fuller. They agreed that a group of nurses and psychiatrists should begin to meet together to reorganize existing approaches to nurse education.[3] To facilitate the process, the NLNE established an official workgroup that would liaise with and report to both the NLNE and the APA: the Committee on Mental Hygiene and Psychiatric Nursing. The workgroup had nine members (Rose Bigler, Elizabeth Bixler, Mary Corchoran, Marian Faber, Daisy Harder, Anna McGibbon, Lena Kranz, Gretchen Nind, Eloise Shields), and May Kennedy was the chair. The committee agreed to conduct a survey of some existing hospital-based schools in an attempt to standardize approaches to curriculum development. Harriet Bailey was engaged to conduct the survey, and she reported her findings in the *American Journal of Nursing* in May 1936. The survey was limited to seven schools (which the APA's Committee on Nursing nominated) in six different states in the north or Midwest and had four objectives:

1.   To determine if the state hospitals for mental disease would offer a basic nursing course.
2.   To observe the organization of the nursing school, its educational program, its application of the nursing service, and the standards of nursing practice resulting therefrom.

3. To determine the clinical resources of nursing education and practice that should be available if a school is to be organized or continued.

4. To offer recommendations along these lines with a view to improvement in the teaching program and ward practice to the end that the mental patient may be better understood and more effectively nursed.[4]

Bailey pointed to the limits of the survey—that it was geographically small and that a single institution could not be said to be representative of the practices across a state with multiple institutions. She recognized that institutions were not homogeneous and subject to the different ideologies and leadership styles of their respective administrators, which immediately signaled a problem at the level of standards and curriculum.[5] Bailey conducted her surveys in thirteen question areas: organization and control of the hospital school; graduate nurse staff; clinical facilities of the hospital; physical facilities of the hospital; health and recreational facilities; student body; classroom instruction; clinical teaching; class and conference evaluation; classrooms and library; and records.

Obviously, these questions were aimed at documenting and developing processes and resources for nurse education, not patient care, but these were not disconnected realms. In her observations and recommendations, Bailey made distinct links between the quality of the educational environment and content, on the one hand, and the intended improvement in patient outcomes on the other. "To conduct a school of nursing," she argued, "the hospital executives and the medical staff should be actively interested in all those aspects of nursing education which affect and hasten the cure and rehabilitation of the patient and increase the effectiveness of nursing care."[6] This required paying attention to the structures and relationships between existing hospital staff and the implications for the graduate nurse. This issue was significantly complicated by the existence of a large untrained attendant workforce and an administration too often lacking enthusiasm for the benefits of further education.

In relation to the attendant workforce, Bailey recognized its dominance and importance but argued that attendants were problematic for patient care due to their substandard training and education. "In all but one institution," she noted, "the attendant group is still the main reliance of the state hospitals especially on the men's division. . . . In only a few instances has any effort been made to establish any educational requirements for employment of this group. . . . Obviously, much more attention should be given to the selection and preparation for service of this group if they are to be charged with the responsibility of administering potent drugs and nursing treatments."[7] It was not that Bailey and her nursing colleagues believed that attendants should become or be called nurses, rather they recognized that the registered nurse workforce shortage, especially in the context of impending war, meant that the care of patients too often fell into the hands of those least well trained. If this situation could not be easily altered, then at the very least attendants should be properly trained.

Bailey made a direct link between trained staff and patient conditions and outcomes, noting that the ratio of what was called "nursing personnel" (meaning both nurses and attendants) to patients in the state hospitals was rarely better than 1:15. Some hospitals had ratios as bad 1:23, even in the chronic disturbed ward. "These figures undoubtedly explain," Bailey lamented, "the very large numbers of untidy, destructive, and assaultive patients in seclusion and restraint on these wards. Moreover, patients in other wards of this hospital were unhappy, uncooperative and resistive, with almost daily accidents to nurses, attendants and other patients—a picture too typical of the old days of minimum care."[8] Bailey's recommendation was that the ratio of nursing personnel to patients should be 1:8, per the APA requirement. But numbers themselves would not be enough to solve the deficiencies in patient care. Bailey argued that more attention needed to be paid to the work and living conditions of attendants in order to "develop a contented, trustworthy and efficient group of workers," and that the "more ambitious" of them should be encouraged to "make up scholastic deficiencies and acquire some of the cultural qualities which are so necessary for success in nursing."[9]

The perceived link between untrained staff and horrendous conditions was a primary concern of nursing leadership, who were desperate to attract more women to psychiatric nursing. This task was made more difficult by the persistence of the hospital training school system, which required the potential psychiatric nurse to commit to living on-site in an often remote location. Thus Bailey's survey also encompassed the living and educational conditions for the student and nursing body associated with each hospital and argued that these needed to be significantly upgraded if a hospital had any hope of attracting young women to live and work there. She stressed the need for a separate residence for the graduate nurses (away from the patients and attendants), good libraries, clean and modern living conditions, and social and recreational activities, overseen "by a person of refinement and interested in young people."[10] Not only would these conditions attract more "respectable" young women, but would address issues of discontent with the working conditions that too often manifested as annoyance and impatience with the patient. Bailey argued that "there are probably no factors more potent in creating a happy, contented, hard-working group of nurses than pleasant living conditions, good food, and reasonable hours for recreation. The hardest and most disagreeable tasks can be faced with courage if one has been fortified by these."[11]

Improving living conditions for resident nurses would not be enough, however. The bulk of Bailey's survey focused on the methods of education employed in each institution, which she found sporadic. Where it was substandard, she lay the blame at the feet of indifferent administrators who failed to recognize the importance of raising educational standards. This indifference stemmed from a general pessimism about the prospects of patient recovery—why pay money for education aimed at better care if the care itself was not going to lead to a cure? This indifference also reflected an indifference to the plight of the mentally ill more broadly—an indifference born of years of lack of funding, increasing patient numbers, and little advance in the science of treatments. Bailey had no patience with these attitudes. She made an explicit link between level of education and patient outcomes when she argued for both purposive and well-planned classroom teaching, as well as an active and interested ward teaching program. Ward teaching in particular provided a unique opportunity for instruction that recognized "that treatment of the patient is a mutual problem of physician and nurses."[12] Hence, a good ward teaching experience was one in which the physician would "stop on ward rounds to hold brief clinics, or in a more informal way to explain the causes of the disordered behavior or the emotional variations and changes so that the nursing procedures may be more intelligently and effectively applied and executed."[13] Combined with case studies, intelligent lectures, well-stocked libraries, and adequately equipped classrooms, this kind of educational program could produce a lively and stimulating environment "with everyone alert and eager to help the patient get well, or to make a happier adjustment to hospital life."[14]

Bailey's survey made two other interesting observations that would become foundational to the development of future programs, and to psychiatric nursing more broadly. These were the ideas that the psychiatric nurse should be employed in all wards regardless of the gender of the patient, and that nurses themselves should be trained to undertake instruction of student nurses. The relationship between gender and psychiatric nursing remained a complex one. In five of the six schools she visited, Bailey noted that "women receive no experience in the care of the male patient," which she felt was a "serious deficiency in the program of education in these schools."[15] As she pointed out, the universal good of the female nurse for all patients in the general hospital was so well accepted as to be a nonissue, and was becoming increasingly linked to the improvement of standards in mental hospitals. She noted that during her site visits, she was directly asked by male patients and physicians "why they didn't have nurses on their wards." These men were referring specifically to the recognizable female graduate registered nurse, not the untrained attendant, but they were referring to them in relation to their gender, not their training. "'They help us to feel more at home' was the reason most frequently given," Bailey explained, and then went on to argue that the female nurse was so necessary because of her very femininity: "Can anyone doubt how unnatural it is for an aging man, accustomed all his life to be looked after at home by mother, wife, or daughters, and in his business by women secretaries and bookkeepers, to be plunged when sick and helpless into an environment where only men, incompetent in nursing, must minister to all his needs?"[16]

The gendered assumptions about both patients and nurses that Bailey made in this report are inseparable from the professionalization agenda of nursing leadership at this time. If the largest workforce in the institutional system was the male attendant, then this was so because he was cheaper to employ than the graduate female nurse. His very presence was a deterrent to women entering the psychiatric nursing workforce because the young woman looking for a new professional pathway had little desire to be associated with the image or reality of the untrained worker. And his presence was a barrier to the expansion of nursing practice areas and to the improvement of both wages and conditions because there was little incentive to invest time and money in creating an alternate workforce. At the same time, for some families thinking of sending their daughters to nursing schools, the overtly sexual nature of some symptoms of mental illnesses were still considered too indelicate for the female practitioner, and this attitude informed Bailey's frequent calls for "refinement" and respectability. These ideas created a set of contradictory claims, however. Nurse leaders like Bailey used gender as a claim to special caring skills for relationships with patients but at the same time argued that these skills were not actually natural and required education and training, which could raise patient outcomes and professional standards. Thus, women claimed legitimacy and authority because they were women and simultaneously claimed professional status based on education. Education then was not enough to be considered a professional psychiatric nurse. Rather, the female nurse was seen to bring something else by virtue of being female that raised her above both the male and the untrained.[17]

The natural extension of a professionalization agenda was that educational instruction should become the purview of the nurse herself. It was obvious to Bailey that the supervisors of residential facilities and patient wards were the domain of the "refined Matron," however the schools she visited had been "slow to realize the advantages of attracting to the principalship of their schools women with superior academic and professional education."[18] While it may be the case that lectures on physiology and anatomy would continue to come from physicians, Bailey argued that nurse instructors could take over some of that work. In fact, in three of the hospitals she visited, "these subjects were taught successfully by nurse instructors who have had special preparation for teaching. These subjects call for many hours in the classroom and should include laboratory periods, to which the busy physician cannot give the required time, and from which he should be relieved."[19] She was, however, quick to recognize the challenges that would need to be overcome before this could become a widespread reality. Minimum standards for nurses as educators would need to be set, and programs for continued education supported by scholarships and prizes. This proactive approach was essential to nursing's continued professionalization, which lagged in comparison to the other psychiatric professions. "The high educational attainments of personnel in other departments only tends to emphasize more clearly the deficiencies in the nursing department,"[20] Bailey lamented. These deficiencies would be best remedied by advanced education outside the hospital school model. For nursing to achieve the same level of respect and intellectual capacity as medicine or social work, the graduate degree was necessary. Given the scope and purpose of the survey, Bailey did not go so far as to say that hospital-based schools should be replaced wholesale with university courses, but she did make some small moves in that direction when she recommended that hospital school students should be encouraged to take courses at universities where possible. "Proximity to a college or a university or other higher institution of learning is an important and valuable factor in stimulating the pursuit of academic and cultural courses by those residing in the hospital," she argued. In the case of any future hospital schools, she encouraged the organizers to consider proximity to higher educational opportunities for nursing staff and students.[21]

If nurses themselves were going to take the lead in the development of psychiatric nursing as an advanced course, then it was necessary for leadership to articulate what form and content that course should take. Accordingly, the second project undertaken by the Committee on Mental Hygiene and Psychiatric Nursing was the development of a curriculum, directed by Anna McGibbon and

Elizabeth Bixler. This project had its origins in the broader work of the NLNE Education Committee, directed by Isabel Stewart, which had sought to articulate objectives and conditions for postgraduate courses across the entirety of nursing. The committee laid out three approaches to developing new knowledge in nurse education: supplementary courses aimed at "rounding out deficiencies" in existing nurse education; reorientation or review courses for continuing education so that the general practice nurse could keep "up to date with newer ideas and methods"; and specialization or advanced courses, aimed at providing an "opportunity for more intensive training on a higher level for nurses who wish to prepare themselves as specialists in one or more of the clinical branches."[22]

Specifically in relation to psychiatry, McGibbon and Bixler envisaged four distinct "units" designed to address each of these areas of need but which would, when taken together, form a lengthy postgraduate course. The four units comprising the course covered orientation to psychiatric nursing; psychiatric nursing; neuropsychiatric nursing of children; and ward administration and principles of teaching. The course was designed to prepare a nurse "for the position of staff nurse, special nurse, head nurse on adult or pediatric wards of a psychiatric hospital, or for a position in other fields of nursing where this specialized knowledge and experience are desired."[23] They published the details of Units I and II in the *American Journal of Nursing* in February 1937, setting out the objectives, suggested time, content, and resources that would be required for each unit. Unit I, lasting only four weeks, was specifically aimed at providing an overview and introduction to psychiatric nursing for the student nurse in order to help her adjust to the type of work and the practice environment, address gaps in her existing education and background, and demonstrate methods of study that would help with this process, as well as to ascertain the student's suitability for this type of work in the long term. In this sense, the orienting nature of the unit was very much aimed at adjusting the student nurse to the clinical environment of the psychiatric hospital or ward, and would therefore "afford the student an opportunity to judge whether she wishes to continue the course."[24]

Unit II, the "Main Course in Psychiatric Nursing," should take at least five months and include six hundred clinical hours, and was aimed at helping the student "to enrich and broaden her clinical background in psychiatric nursing."[25] Rather than focus solely on structure, the course also outlined some objectives for specific content, which were drawn partially from the results of a survey of fifteen schools of nursing that currently offered postgraduate courses through an affiliated mental hospital. These objectives imagined the role of the nurse as an active user of scientific knowledge for the benefit of both the patient and the nurse herself. For example, not only would the nurse taking this course "develop an understanding of the mental mechanisms and motivations basic to an interpretation of human behavior," she would also learn "to depict the patient as a total personality" and to adapt her practices to meet the patient's physical, mental, and emotional needs.[26] In doing so, she would draw on the work that nurses had already done to articulate the connection between mental and physical illness, as well as on new theories within psychiatry itself. The course should therefore present "the contributions of the various schools of psychiatric thought" so that they could be evaluated for their usefulness to the individual patient. This development of a "psychiatric attitude" could then be applied by the nurse across multiple practice settings including "the general hospital, private duty, and public health nursing."[27] Nowhere in the suggested content for the course do the words "mental hygiene" appear, yet the concept is there in principle. Objectives 4 and 5 are explicitly related to the social and environmental contexts of mental health and illness—"social disorganization (crime, delinquency, alcoholism et cetera)"—to which the nurse must be attuned, as well as emphasizing "the importance of mental disease as a public health problem and the responsibility of the nurse in furthering a mental health program in the community."[28] To enhance understanding in this area, the course should include thirty hours of work in sociology, which would help the student appreciate social and environmental issues as "precipitating factors in mental disease." These should be combined with case histories that "may be used as illustrations of the theory that man is, in part, the product of social forces."[29] Of course, no five-month course could do justice to this complex theory, so it was envisioned that the first two units of study would be combined with two more units aimed at child neuropsychiatry and administration and teaching.

These extra units were not published in the *American Journal of Nursing*, however, and when the NLNE published its updated *Curriculum Guide for Schools of Nursing* in 1937, there was no mention of a postgraduate option for psychiatric nursing. The curriculum guide did include descriptions of courses that would introduce nurses to concepts from sociology and psychology, as articulated above, as well as a course on "Social Problems in the Nursing Service," but these were all designed to be integrated into the undergraduate nursing curriculum. This remained the stance of the NLNE in relation to psychiatry—the curriculum guide included provisions for a twelve-week course of study in psychiatric nursing that would introduce the undergraduate student to the basics of psychiatric knowledge and its applications for patient care, including its importance for all of nursing and its social and public health implications,

but there was no formal move toward postgraduate specialty by the NLNE at
this stage.[30]

Working with the APA

The extensive suggestions for revised curriculums developed by McGibbon and
Bixler were presented separately to the new chair of the APA's Committee on
Nursing, George Stevenson, in October 1937 during a meeting with members of
both the ANA and the NLNE in New York City. They were published in the
American Journal of Psychiatry in 1939 as "Psychiatric Nursing Education: Recommended Standards and Curricula for Undergraduate General Nursing
Courses in Psychiatric Hospitals, Affiliate and Postgraduate Courses in Psychiatric Nursing."[31] Stevenson introduced the article with a recognition of the part-
nership with the NLNE and the comment that this was "the first major revision
since standards were set by the American Psychiatric Association in 1923."[32]
The most extensive of these were the plans for the two types of postgraduate
courses that would be run by schools of nursing with psychiatric affiliations,
indicating a general interest in moving away from the psychiatric hospital-run
school of nursing. The Advanced Postgraduate Course was designed to be not
less than twelve months "and may be longer."[33] As McGibbon and Bixler had
set out, it would include units on the psychiatric aspects of public health nursing, child psychiatry, teaching, and administration, and was designed specifically "for the special training of the nurse who plans a definite career in the
psychiatric field."[34] The sticking point for this type of course, however, and for
the development of advanced psychiatric nursing more generally, was that the
accreditation for these courses was still to be issued by the APA.

While Stevenson's article spelled out that any psychiatric hospital offer-
ing general nursing needed to do so in association with the State Nurses'
Board, this was not the case for the psychiatric specialties. For many in nursing leadership this was nonnegotiable: the accreditation of nursing courses
needed to be the purview of the NLNE. This insistence conflicted with the
reality of psychiatric nursing education. Schools of nursing were barely
equipped to teach psychiatry, and needed to create a cadre of educators who
were qualified to do so. Yet this could not happen without more advanced
courses to train those educators. The efforts of the APA were also undermined
by the continued poor quality of existing hospital-based graduate and affiliate
courses. The NLNE's Committee on Curriculum reported at the 1939 conference their own dissatisfaction with the current state of APA-certified courses,
arguing that "the distinction between the various types of courses is not carefully drawn in practice. . . . A certificate presented by a nurse may have little

relationship to her competence for a position which requires advanced preparation."[35] At the 1940 NLNE conference, May Kennedy was forced to report that at the most recent APA conference she had heard numerous complaints from superintendents about the courses, including a lack of enrolments, a lack of enthusiasm for psychiatric work, and their own dwindling interest in continuing to provide affiliate courses for nurses.[36]

While Kennedy agreed with the assessments of existing courses, she urged the NLNE leadership not to throw the proverbial baby out with the bathwater. She supported Stevenson's call for the appointment of a full-time consultant to try and work out a systemic solution to the problems, and pointed out that he had long been an advocate for graduate courses as the model for psychiatric nursing education. In 1934 Stevenson had presented a paper at the annual meeting of the APA where he addressed the historical practice of the state hospital-based training school. He argued that the system, while the best that was available at the time, was now inadequate and had presented a false economy. "A training school properly conducted," he stated, "probably cost as much or more than to staff with graduate nurses."[37] In attempting to economize, the superintendent did a disservice to both his patients, who were not exposed to the best care possible, and to student nurses, who were not receiving an adequate education. For Stevenson, the answer lay with general nurses' graduate training in psychiatry: "The nurse in our mental hospital should be thoroughly equipped with the ordinary or general training so that she may do justice to all the physical features, but in addition she should understand more of the workings of the human mind, and the influence of environmental and emotional stresses. . . . And even more than this, she needs to know the possibilities of effecting improvement through psychotherapy, and to know the part she should be able to play in the treatment scheme."[38]

Stevenson's call for graduate education then was in part a reflection of the concern of professional psychiatry that institutions become more than mere warehouses, and signaled the growing impact of psychodynamic therapies on psychiatric practice more broadly. Significantly, Stevenson argued that the control of that education should now be turned over to nursing itself: "The nursing profession should attempt to set standards for its own professional requirements . . . and should probably have some voice in saying whether or not any particular school should or should not train nurses."[39] It was not simply enough to upskill attendants. Rather, nursing organizations needed to "arrange such affiliations or post graduate courses" as were necessary to ensure that the general nurse could be adequately prepared for work in psychiatry.[40] To attempt any less was unacceptable "if the patient's need is our first consideration as it should be."[41]

Stevenson felt that there was still a need for the attendant, but the standards for these needed to be raised at the same time as the registered nurse advanced in her knowledge and skill. Without these advances, both the patient, and the profession, would suffer: "The unrecovered cases are simply an indication of our treatment failures, and a challenge to our still greater therapeutic and nursing efforts. In fairness to the patient as well as in fairness to ourselves only the best nursing service should be available."[42]

Some of Stevenson's concerns were shared by other psychiatric leaders, who began to argue more overtly for the need for graduate general nurses to pursue psychiatry as a specialty. In 1937 five psychiatrists, including Adolf Meyer, William A. White, and William Menninger, published a collection of short pieces in the *American Journal of Nursing* about the importance of postgraduate work in psychiatric nursing. In these articles they argued for a more highly trained professional who could deal with both the physical and psychological effects of illness in both the general and the mental hospital, but who specifically had the intellect and personality to more actively participate in therapeutic practices within the psychiatric institution or ward.[43] In 1938 Menninger was part of the NLNE's convention in Kansas City, Missouri, and he gave a lengthy paper entitled "Psychiatry in Nursing Education."[44] In this paper, Menninger argued that psychiatric nursing was the foundation of all nursing, largely because the distinction between mind and body when it came to illness was a false one. Therefore, psychiatry had implications for nursing across the spectrum, including for the self-awareness and maturity of the nurse herself. More than this, however, Menninger argued that the nurse with advanced training could and should be an active part of the therapeutic program. A value of psychiatry to the nurse, he argued, "is its opportunity for her to make herself a therapist rather than merely a doctor's handmaiden. . . . Psychiatry can teach the nurse that she herself automatically becomes 'medicine' for her patient."[45]

Stevenson continued to argue in the same vein in his work with the NLNE. Also in 1938, he explicitly recognized the need for further education in psychiatry "so that new treatments can be given by intelligent and skilled nurses. The psychiatrist will be greatly handicapped in his scientific work if he does not have qualified nurses to assist him."[46] However, he argued that if this type of nurse were to emerge, it would require centralized coordination through the appointment of a single person "in some national organization who would devote all her time to mental hygiene and psychiatric work. Her chief function for some time would be to interest nurses in general and directors of schools of nursing, in the hope that they will see the importance of all nurses being prepared to care for the mental as well as the physical aspects of illness. This nurse would also assist administrators in mental hospitals in planning affiliate and graduate courses, setting standards, and procuring qualified faculty members."[47] Stevenson envisaged this person as a kind of consultant—a nurse who would liaise between the APA, NLNE, and various schools of nursing. When he was elected president of the APA in 1940, it fell to his successor as chair of the Committee on Nursing, Charles Fitzpatrick, to make this idea a reality.

Nurse Consultants and the Rockefeller Foundation

In his 1941 report to the APA Executive Committee, Fitzpatrick wrote that it was time for the APA to secure funds to formally address the long-running nursing education standards problem, and he recommended approaching the Rockefeller Foundation.[48] The Rockefeller Foundation had a long history of funding psychiatric work, including the earlier mental hygiene movement and the evaluation of schools of nursing. Fitzpatrick and Arthur Ruggles, who was now the secretary of the APA, met with Alan Gregg, the director of medical services for the Rockefeller Foundation, in February 1941 in New York. All three men were cognizant of the many reasons that psychiatric nurses were in such short supply, given the requirements for nurse education and the impact of impending war. They were therefore keen to address problems with the attendant workforce as well—not to replace nursing, but as a complementary measure. As Fitzpatrick explained to Gregg, "The present defense program has, of course, accentuated the deficit and is slowly but surely starving the civilian hospitals . . . a partial solution lies in the training of psychiatric attendants so that they can carry on some of the simpler procedures which are now engaging the time of nurses."[49] Fitzpatrick noted that there were at least eighty-seven institutions giving training of some sort to attendants but that there was no standardization or accreditation of these courses. He argued that the APA should have some say over the way that attendant training was organized and accredited, and that the motivation for this endeavor was, ultimately, improved patient care. "I have long since come down out of the clouds," he declared, "and realize that men and women must be trained, call them by whatever title we may, for there is work that must be done and patients must be cared for."[50] He was quick to stress, however, that whatever efforts were made in this area must be done in collaboration with nursing: "Should such courses for the training of attendants be approved in any way by the Council, they should be worked out in detail in collaboration with the National League of Nursing Education and some provision should be made in the various states for the licensing of such psychiatric attendants."[51] This was an overt recognition of nurses' concerns about their relationship with attendants.

After more meetings later in 1941, Gregg finally agreed to funding for a nurse consultant, writing in his diary, "Told Fitzpatrick, after discussion of the state of psychiatric nursing, that I was willing to have the APA put in an application for a grant not to exceed $10000 for a year. The situation both for nurses and orderlies is aggravated by the wartime demands, but will remain for a long time a serious and embarrassing difficulty in the work of mental hospitals."[52] For his part, having long worked with schools and associations of nursing through the Rockefeller Foundation's Division of Medical Services, Gregg was aware of the emerging power of professional nursing associations, and Fitzpatrick convinced him that he was confident of nursing support, stating that the "appointee would work in close conjunction and collaboration with the National League of Nursing Education, and I have been assured by Miss May Kennedy, Chairman of the Committee on Psychiatric Nursing of that organization, that her committee would collaborate willfully and fully in this project."[53]

After much deliberation about potential candidates, in July 1942 the APA appointed Laura Wood Fitzsimmons as its inaugural nurse consultant. Alan Gregg met her in New York in mid-1942 and noted the following about her in his diary: "She is Virginia born and bred, trained at Walter Reed Hosp. and later a supervising nurse there; was in the Army three years with service at Fort Sheridan and in Manila; 2½ years at Gallinger Hosp. in Washington; and then 3½ years at Payne Whitney during which time secured as of 1938 her B. Sc. at Columbia in nursing ed; was subsequently supt. of nursing at St. Elizabeths Hosp."[54] This was an impressive pedigree. As one of the country's largest psychiatric hospitals, St. Elizabeths was also home to a number of innovative psychiatrists, including Superintendent Wilfred Overholser who was a noted psychoanalyst and colleague of Harry Stack Sullivan. Gregg was also impressed by Fitzsimmons's personal qualities, noting that "she seems well balanced in point of helping people and with level-headed understanding, simple and effective methods of procedure."[55] This pragmatic approach was important to Gregg, whose interest in psychiatry was much less ideological then it was practical. In their meeting, he explained to Fitzsimmons that his idea of success would be an increasing number of requests for her advice coming from various mental hospitals. This reflected the Rockefeller's focus on funding projects that had immediate impact, that were supportive of primary care personnel, and that would lead to long-term, self-sustaining projects with a focus on measurable improvements for staff and patients.

Fitzsimmons's first task for the APA was to conduct a survey of the state of the field, and she did this through written questionnaires and personal visits. She traveled across the United States and Canada and documented the state of

psychiatric nursing and attendant workforces as well as systems for nurse education, which culminated in a report delivered to the APA and the Rockefeller
Foundation in June 1944. She made a number of observations and recommendations as a result of this survey that were always tempered by a recognition
of the severe staffing and educational shortages caused by the war, which had
consumed so many nursing positions.

Concerned with approaching the issue from all angles, Fitzsimmons made
eight major recommendations for the postwar period. These argued for the need
for public awareness campaigns about mental illness; an increase of funds into
mental health so as to facilitate better standards of hours, wages, and conditions
for workers; a uniform system of training for attendants; the development of uniform standards of care for patients; more clinical placements in mental health
for student nurses; improving schools of nursing associated with mental hospitals; the creation of degree-level postgraduate courses in mental health; specific
professional recognition for mental health nurses; and the organization of mental
health staff under a director of nursing.[56]

None of these recommendations are particularly surprising; they reflect the
debates that both nurses and psychiatrists had been having for some time. But
in her private letters to the Rockefeller Foundation Fitzsimmons identifies other,
thornier, issues. In a long letter to Gregg in 1943, she noted the issues facing
inpatient psychiatric care on a number of fronts. Personnel shortages remained
the most immediate problem, which had a long history due to lack of federal
funding and had been exacerbated by "the poor salaries paid in mental hospitals, the long hours and poor living conditions [that] have not been conducive
to attracting personnel."[57] The lack of funding for institutions also had serious
implications for patient care. Fitzsimmons noted that the financial logic needed
to change: now that treatment options had expanded to be actively therapeutic
and not merely custodial, more resources needed to be appropriated.[58] This was
not just a hospital management problem but one of quality of care. Patient outcomes could not change until the quality of education for personnel improved.
Fitzsimmons noted that postgraduate courses were almost nonexistent, and
reflected to some extent the lack of psychiatric or mental health content in the
undergraduate nursing curriculum. Without this content, there was no pathway
from undergraduate general nursing to graduate specialist psychiatric nursing.
Despite these many challenges, Fitzsimmons remained cautiously optimistic:
"In conclusion, it may be said that fortunately the picture is not always distress-
ing. There are mental hospitals where all patients receive the benefit of a fine
type of physical and psychological nursing care, where restraint is unknown
and happiness prevails. When such conditions are observed, especially at this

critical period, one is prone to believe that the superintendents of such institutions are not only physicians, but also magicians."[59]

In the absence of magic, however, real-world solutions were required. One
of the recommendations from Fitzsimmons's report that was most quickly realized was her call for uniform standards of patient care and attendant training.
As well as conducting surveys and writing reports, Fitzsimmons produced a
370-page training manual for attendants. The manual covered all aspects of
patient care, from the most technical and mundane to high-level therapeutic
techniques. It had a specific focus on the day-to-day tasks, which were presented
not just as the basic requirements for patient care but as therapeutic opportunities. The Rockefeller Foundation funded the production and dissemination of
the manual and the first edition completely sold out, with requests to the APA
for copies continuing for some time.

While a success in its own right, Fitzsimmons's work on attendants had a
broader purpose. She had sought to differentiate the nature of attendant or aide
work from that of nurses and establish actual standards for education and training of aide staff, over whom nurses would then have control. She was impatient to establish the courses by which nurses could attain the qualifications
necessary to take on a greater leadership role within institutions. After the delivery of the attendant manual, she moved her focus more intently to the development of university courses for psychiatric nursing. As Gregg noted in his diary
in June 1945, "Mrs. F-S says she wants next year's emphasis to be spent princi-
pally on the development of postgraduate courses in psychiatric nursing. . . .
The desperately urgent need is for registered nurses with thorough postgraduate training in psychiatric nursing who can teach students and students of
nursing on affiliation."[60]

If there was to be any meaningful development of psychiatric nursing skills,
then skilled nurses were needed to teach the next generation. Fitzsimmons wrote
publicly about these issues. Her article "University Controlled Advanced Clinical Programs in Psychiatric Nursing" was published in the *American Journal
of Nursing* in December 1944, and had been read and revised by Gregg before
she submitted it. In this article, she set out a clear rationale for the development
of university-based courses that would elevate the profession into the realm of
academic scholarship and research as well as provide leaders and administrators into the future. She made the pointed observation that "for years we have
talked about the need for a well-rounded program of nurse education yet, while
preaching this doctrine, year after year hundreds of nurses have been graduated
from schools of nursing without having had any experience in the field of

psychiatric nursing while psychiatry claims over 50 percent of the hospital beds of the nation."[61]

Fitzsimmons summed up the existing situation for her readers by explaining that nothing could change until there were adequately trained instructors, and this was her justification for university-based courses: "Little can be done to advance psychiatric training at an undergraduate level until more key people are available to direct, instruct, and supervise these programs. The need for knowledge of psychiatric nursing has been so generally recognized that requests for student affiliations in all areas of the country are far in excess of the courses and nurse instructors available."[62] This was a complex problem impacted by the intricacies of federal funding. It was one thing to want courses; it was another thing entirely to make them happen. In a letter to Gregg in November 1944, Fitzpatrick stated that Fitzsimmons had been successful at persuading four universities "to set up graduate instruction to meet this need and two others are in the process of developing such courses in 1945."[63] These were not, however, the extensive graduate courses that nurses were imagining; rather, they were short-term (three-month) certificate courses for graduate registered nurses, but these early successes were nevertheless the stepping stones for much larger changes that would emerge after World War II.

At the same time as the APA had been attempting to address the issue of nursing education, the Menninger brothers had been working on approaches to the training of attendants. Despite the growing recommendations of the various NLNE and APA projects, and the recognition that educated nurses were better for patient outcomes, psychiatrists continued to push for the expansion of the attendant workforce and for the improvement of standards of attendant training as the cheapest and fastest way to meet their institutional workforce needs. In 1947 Karl Menninger wrote to the Rockefeller Foundation about his idea for developing an attendant training program at their clinic in Topeka, Kansas. The world-famous Menninger brothers were central figures in mental health at this time and impossible to ignore. In the leadup to World War II, William Menninger was appointed the chief psychiatric consultant to the surgeon general. After the war, William established and led the Group for the Advancement of Psychiatry from 1946, and became president of the APA from 1948 to 1949 while still running the Menninger Clinic with his brother Karl.

The Menningers were looking to start a school for the training of psychiatric aides within the Veterans Administration (VA) system in Kansas. The primary objective, as Karl Menninger explained to Robert Morrison, the new director of medical services at the Rockefeller Foundation, was "to try and improve the quality of care given by aides to patients."[64] Interestingly, Menninger did not see aides as merely performing simple tasks, which would free up nurses and which Fitzpatrick had argued for in the earlier nurse consultant program. Rather, as he had previously argued in relation to nurses, Menninger saw aides as essential members of the therapeutic team. In relation to the project at the VA, Menninger did not appear particularly sympathetic to the cause of nurses themselves. Rather, he argued that the training of psychiatric aides needed to happen regardless of whatever nurses were doing, and that it needed to happen quickly. As he explained to Morrison, "I do not want to swerve from my determination to do something in the direction of aide training and I feel that we doctors must not relinquish this to such initiative as may develop in the nursing profession."[65]

The Rockefeller Foundation was supportive to a point—they recognized the importance of the aide, and the need for a fully trained "sub professional" group. But they did not go so far as to suggest that this project could or should happen without the input of nurses. For his part, Menninger knew that the idea would meet resistance in some form from nursing—he admitted as much to the foundation early in the process when he noted, "There is a strong emotional opposition on the part of some nurse leaders."[66] It was hardly an emotional opposition, however. It was, in fact, as the foundation noted, "largely because the nurses fear an infringement of their rights and status."[67] The foundation listened to nurses on this point.

As such, the Rockefeller Foundation expressed initial hesitance to fund the Menninger project. "I do have some grounds for feeling," Morrison wrote in his Rockefeller diary, "that the Menninger brothers sometimes promise things, the implications of which they have not fully thought through."[68] In this project, it was the implications for nursing, and the strength of the opposition, that the Menningers had not considered. Morrison made some notes from a phone conversation with William Menninger early in 1949 in which he wrote that Menninger "would be willing to substitute a nurse for a psychiatrist as director of the school but fears that would not entirely meet all the objections."[69] Indeed it did not. The project did not in fact get off the ground at the Menningers' preferred site of the Winter VA Hospital in Topeka because the nursing staff there ultimately refused to facilitate a training program for aides over which they would not have complete control. The Menningers were able to establish their training school for psychiatric aides at the Topeka State Hospital instead. Here the nurses were less of a force to be reckoned with because the state hospital was not at the time affiliated with any nursing school. This meant there were no nurse-led standards for education or accreditation of courses already in place,

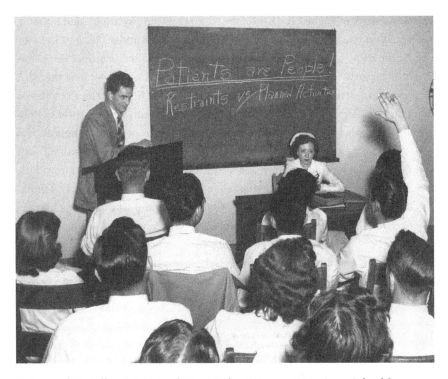

Dr. Bernard H. Hall and Registered Nurse Esther L. Lazaro, Menninger School for Psychiatric Aides, Topeka, Kansas, 1949. Photo courtesy of the Rockefeller Archives Center, Record Group 1.1, Series 219: Kansas.

and the Menningers could therefore do as they liked with the $75,000 the Rockefeller Foundation eventually gave them.

The Menningers quickly established a school for psychiatric aides at the Topeka State Hospital. The school ran for a few years under the direction of a psychiatrist, Dr. Bernard Hall, who worked with nurse Esther Lazaro, associate director of the school and supervisor of clinical training.

In 1951, however, Hall reported to the foundation that the school was closing, and they discontinued funding. In his diary, Morrison noted, "My guess is that H [Hall] has succumbed to pressure from the nurses who feel the competition of well-trained psychiatric aides. It seems to have been an increasing problem to find out just where the highly trained psychiatric aide would fit into the administrative picture in mental hospitals."[70]

In the meantime, Laura Fitzsimmons had left her role at the APA in order to take up a role as chief of psychiatric nursing for the VA.[71] With continued funding from the Rockefeller Foundation, the APA employed two more full-time nurse consultants, Lela Anderson and Dorothy Clarke. They both continued the important work of negotiating the relationship between psychiatry and nursing, but noted increasing resistance to their efforts. Clarke undertook another survey for the APA, which was published in 1950, but it failed to attract responses from the majority of schools of nursing, who perhaps no longer saw the APA as the authoritative or answerable body in the field. In 1951 the Rockefeller Foundation's nursing field officer, Mary Elizabeth Tenant, wrote a letter to Robert Morrison in which she was bluntly scathing of the repeated attempts at data collection with no real outcome. She suggested that the nurse consultant program was now a redundant approach and a duplication of time and effort. Further, she argued that there was extremely competent leadership at the national level in relation to nursing education in psychiatry, and it was past time for psychiatrists to hand over the reins to the ANA, NLNE, and the National Organization of Public Health Nurses.[72] Tenant's comments were a recognition of the work that was already happening through these organizations, and reflected the impact that changes in federal legislation were beginning to have on the capacity of nursing to organize university-based courses.

The NLNE Curriculum Committee

In reality, the only body with any control over the establishment of nursing courses in universities was the accrediting body, the NLNE. The NLNE had a committee devoted to the development and revision of nursing school curriculums, and it was through this body that nurses began to agitate for real system-level change. Their arguments were given a boost in 1943, when the federal government passed the Bolton Act, a $1.2 million appropriation designed to address the shortage of nurses that had been made painfully apparent by World War II. The Act provided funding for universities and colleges to develop advanced courses for graduate nurses aimed at providing administrative and educational leadership, and for the development of specific clinical specialties.[73] In a roundtable discussion on psychiatric nursing at the 1942 convention of the NLNE, May Kennedy continued to advocate for the integration of psychiatric nursing across the undergraduate curriculum, partly because she believed mental health could not be separated from physical health and that therefore all nurses needed to know something about psychiatry.[74] This point of view gained some traction—by 1944, 54 percent of U.S. nursing schools offered a "basic experience" in psychiatric nursing.[75] But it was also the case that specialization was required not just for patient care but for the type of education that Kennedy herself desired. When the nursing education consultant with the U.S. Public Health Service, Eugenia Spalding, participated at the same roundtable, she made the point that one way out of psychiatric nursing's current circular logic was to avail itself of Bolton Act funds and create its own graduate courses aimed at the creation of psychiatric nursing as a clinical specialty. The lure of funds was the final spur to decisive NLNE action.

In 1945 the NLNE's Special Committee on Postgraduate Clinical Courses and its Subcommittee on Psychiatric Nursing published the second pamphlet in its series "Courses in Clinical Nurses for Graduate Nurses": *An Advanced Course in Psychiatric Nursing.*[76] The committee consisted of five people: Anna McGibbon (chair), Elizabeth Bixler, Laura Fitzsimmons, Eloise Shields, and Elizabeth Porter ex officio as chair of the broader committee on postgraduate clinical nursing courses. The pamphlet drew explicitly on the earlier curriculum work that McGibbon and Bixler had already done for the NLNE and APA, and was informed by Fitzsimmons's work as the APA nursing consultant and her focus on advanced courses within universities. The introduction to the pamphlet clearly spelled out that what was being advocated now was the creation of psychiatric nursing as a specialty that built on psychiatric material that had been included in undergraduate nursing courses: "The proposed course must constitute a part of an advanced program in nursing in an accredited university or college or be approved for credit by that university or college. The proposed course represents advanced study and experience in the field of psychiatric nursing arranged for the nurse who wishes to become a specialist, as differentiated from the basic course which should be part of the professional preparation of all nurses."[77] With this statement, the document mandated both integration *and* specialization, and signified the importance of psychiatric concepts for all nurse education. The difference between a basic course and specialist training, however, was clearly articulated in the "Purpose of the Course," where the authors noted that the time allotted to psychiatry and mental health in the basic course was insufficient for the development of specific abilities afforded by specialization. These included the ability to understand subtleties in symptom expression, the recognition of the motivations for patient behavior, and anticipating changes in that behavior. Moreover, the nurse who had completed the basic course may know what some approaches to patients were, and that there may be different requirements for different patients, but she would not have progressed so far as to understand the significance of her own attitudes or behaviors and their impact on the patient. Therefore, the recommended qualifications for admission were not just evidence of completion of "an acceptable basic professional course in psychiatric nursing" but also that the applicants should be "intellectually mature and emotionally stable individuals who have demonstrated fitness for continuing to work in this field."[78]

An Advanced Course in Psychiatric Nursing made the unusual step of setting out a number of clinical examples where the benefits of specialization and
maturity would be evident. In these examples, the authors explicitly articulated
both the negative and positive effects the nurse could have on direct patient care,
and in doing so presented principles of clinical practice that went far beyond
basic nursing tasks. For example, the basically trained nurse would be more
likely to resort to seclusion of a disturbed patient "because she lacks the experience, techniques and understanding which would enable her to substitute a
superior plan of care."[79] In contrast, the nurse with advanced education would
be better able to "evaluate the total situation" and less likely to resort to seclusion as a first measure because she would have been trained in alternatives and
in methods for gaining the cooperation of patients. She would have better understanding of the patient as a whole, of their motivations and of their needs, rather
than basing her actions on fear or distrust. The significance of the relationship
between the advanced nurse and the patient featured in a number of other examples, including her ability to understand the changing moods of the depressed
and suicidal, observing them in an unobtrusive way, and using explanation and
reassurance rather than restraints.[80] Significantly, the nurse with advanced preparation would be more aware of her own background and emotional baggage,
and would learn techniques to avoid projection, attachment, and inappropriate
mothering of the patient at the same time as she would learn to be less controlling and less judgmental of the difficult or noncompliant patient.[81]

The authors of the pamphlet suggested that this highly reflective and nearly
autonomous practitioner could only be created through a genuine commitment
to a lengthy course of not less than nine months, with significant clinical experience based as much as possible on intensive case work in American Medical
Association-accredited hospitals.[82] This particular note was an interesting break
from the APA, which did not rate a mention in the entire document. Rather, it
was suggested that the student should work closely with other professionals like
the social worker or the public health nurse to experience the various settings
within which the mental health patient may be found; that is, not just the long-
term custodial institution. The type of practice being articulated in this document was recovery oriented, aimed at working with patients through an acute
inpatient phase of illness but in such a way that the goal was discharge from
hospital and a return to home or community settings where some level of normal functioning would be possible. In this sense, the course was intrinsically
situated in the social and environmental context of postwar America.

In particular, the NLNE's vision for the advanced course reflected the particular social and political influence of World War II. The fifth objective, for

example, was dedicated entirely to articulating the importance of the nurse in the repatriation effort, and in the preparation of both families and returned service people with physical and mental injuries. To do so, the nurse would need to understand "the importance of psychological factors in the rehabilitation of service men and women" and "the psychological effect of crippling physical disability."[83] She would need to know about rehabilitation programs for veterans, and to work in both the inpatient and outpatient space as part of a holistic team with the social worker. For the veteran's family, she would need to be able to explain the psychic effects of war and be able to teach them a "healthful attitude toward war-injured individuals" who may be "tense, irritable, sensitive to noises, emotionally labile."[84] The nurse also needed to be able to deal with problems of adjustment for the returned or rejected service men and women as they struggled with new illnesses, tried to find new types of work, or simply adjust to peace time.

These problems were situated in broader social changes and concerns about postwar poverty and the creation of a robust and resilient society. To this end, a great deal of the course content was dedicated to outpatient work and to providing holistic care in the community setting. The techniques and skills the nurse would need to undertake this work drew heavily on nursing's earlier engagement with mental hygiene, which now made an overt reappearance. The "Sub Unit" on "Social and Community Aspects of Psychiatric Care" had the central objective of developing "comprehensive knowledge of the social significance of mental disease and of community facilities for promoting social adjustments to enable participation in the improvement of the mental health of individuals, families and communities."[85] The content of the course was aimed at developing the nurses' "understanding of the emotional adjustments of adults to lack of financial security, unemployment or sporadic employment, lack of opportunity for satisfying work, or loss of social status," as well as "the emotional adjustments of children to poverty, bad housing, unemployed parents."[86] In the same way that nurses had written about mental hygiene, the well-rounded psychiatric nurse should be skilled in history-taking and needed to learn how to evaluate experiences in the person's early life that "may have pointed to psychoses" and how to suggest "adjustments which might have prevented the illness."[87] She would need to know how to undertake home visits and look for circumstances in the environment or in the person's relationships that may be triggers to illness, and she would need "a comprehensive knowledge of preventive methods, particularly in the area of child care."[88]

Despite this focus on social and community settings, the advanced course was intended to be firmly grounded in the latest psychiatric theory and method.

The overarching objective was the "attainment of a comprehensive knowledge of psychiatric disorders and of recent developments in scientific care and treatment."[89] To this end, the nurse would be educated in the "structure of personality as taught by different schools of psychiatric thought" and would have a comprehensive "understanding of the dynamics of human behavior."[90] She would need to understand the physiology of mental disease, the flow of cause and effect between the brain and the body, and thus be well versed in all the methods of psychosomatic treatment. These treatments ranged from shock therapy, "fever treatment," and neurosurgical procedures to pharmacology and "psychotherapy (including psychoanalysis)."[91] The course outline did not go so far as to say that the nurse should be applying these therapies herself, but it did specify that she would learn them through lectures and case studies, and that she would learn to assist with them through extensive clinical experience. The overall goal of the course, therefore, was to create a nurse who was capable of "analyzing complex and varied psychiatric nursing situations so that all significant factors are recognized and interpreted" and "planning and executing skillfully a related program of nursing."[92]

Toward Professional Power

The debates and activities that nurses and psychiatrists engaged in throughout the 1940s spoke to the increasing awareness of the significance of the nurse in mental health care and treatment. It was clear to all concerned that the mental health of the nation depended on educated and skilled practitioners, and that improvements in standards of care and curriculums were needed to improve both the image of psychiatry and the actual outcomes for patients. Hospital-based psychiatrists were pragmatists, and willing to attack the problem from all angles, which meant addressing the issue of the unskilled attendant as much as it did supporting the registered nurse. At times the goals of psychiatrists were in tandem with those of nurses, but at times they clashed, which was particularly evident when nursing leadership began to pursue a strong professionalization agenda. While improvements in patient care and a contribution to the social project of mental health were stated objectives of the committees and projects undertaken by nurses themselves, there was often an underlying context of a push for power. Knowledge would be essential for a clinical specialty and for patient care but the political and social significance of psychiatry in the postwar period gave nursing leadership the impetus to expand its professional agenda, which was the ultimate control of both psychiatric nursing education and practice under the auspices of nurses themselves.

While some nurses advocated for continued relationships with psychiatrists, nursing leadership's impatience with psychiatric control came to a head during World War II. At the same time, the debates within nursing itself about whether psychiatric education should take place at the undergraduate or graduate level revealed the profession to be at a crossroads. Was nursing leadership prepared to take the leap into clinical specialties? Did nursing have the infrastructure and the talent to do so? The Bolton Act had been hugely successful in stabilizing the basic nurse workforce during wartime, as well as creating the Nurse Cadet Corps. But it had not created a cadre of nurse educators who could take the place of psychiatrists, and it had not created the ability to establish widespread graduate courses within universities. While a few short-term graduate courses were in effect by the end of the war, these were not the intensive university-based courses that many in nursing's leadership imagined. In advocating for psychiatry as an advanced specialty, which could be run by nurses themselves, leadership needed to acknowledge that they did not yet have the cadre of highly educated and suitably qualified nurses who could teach those courses at a participating university. Similarly, as Fitzsimmons had revealed in her work for the Rockefeller Foundation, universities themselves were not yet in a position to offer, and were not even particularly interested in, those programs. At the end of the day, the question was always: Who would pay for them?

The Bolton Act expired with the end of World War II, and this meant the end of appropriations for training stipends for individual nurses. But the end of the war also bought new opportunities. Individual scholarships for graduate education would be provided by the GI Bill (1944), and, for psychiatric nurses, structural funding for new program development became available with the passing of the National Mental Health Act (1946) and the establishment of the National Institute of Mental Health (1948). It was through these structures that nursing leadership for psychiatry could be centralized, as Mary Tenant had suggested. But the question remained about who would be qualified to run and teach these new programs, and what exactly they would be teaching. Chapter 4 explores the different ways that nurses themselves attempted to answer these questions.

"We Called It 'Talking with Patients'"

Interpersonal Relations and the Idea of Nurses as Therapists

The year 1948 was an important one for American psychiatry. The new National Institute of Mental Health (NIMH) began to make funds available for research and advanced training. William Menninger appeared on the cover of *Time* magazine for an article entitled "Are You Always Worrying?" William's older brother Karl wrote the preface to journalist Albert Deutsch's scathing exposé of mental hospitals, *The Shame of the States*. And psychiatric nurses found themselves represented on the big screen in the film adaptation of Mary Jane Ward's 1946 novel *The Snake Pit*. Based partially on the author's experiences at Rockland State Hospital in New York, the book and film were received as "a cryptic but trenchant revelation of a crying need for better facilities for mental care."[1] These exposés highlighted the twin evils of understaffing and overcrowding and often portrayed nurses as complicit and sometimes abusive. Professional nursing was not unaware of this portrayal, and it rankled. A review of the film *The Snake Pit* published in the *American Journal of Nursing* argued that the movie portrayed nurses unfairly and did not consider the true efforts that they had taken to improve patient conditions in the preceding years. At the same time, the editor reminded nurses that the popularity of the movie would require both a concerted public relations effort on the part of mental health professionals and continued work from nurses in order to improve relationships with both patients and the public. The reviewer argued that "with *The Snake Pit* goading the public conscience, nurses have an excellent opportunity to articulate leadership in building a better world."[2]

This chapter explores this articulation of leadership throughout the 1950s as nurses availed themselves of new funds from the NIMH to take charge of their own education and practice. There was no single approach to this new program of work, which now began to develop as a clinical specialty. Rather, a new generation of emerging nurse leaders were encouraged to develop programs that reflected their own philosophical or theoretical approach, and their individual perceptions of the needs of both the profession and the patient. The way in which graduate programs developed in the 1950s reflected the dynamic and eclectic nature of psychiatric theory and practice at this time and the therapeutic problems with which it engaged. Despite these differences, often specific to place or institution, running through nursing debates and knowledge in the 1950s and 1960s was a thread centered around interpersonal theory and its significance for the nurse-patient relationship. Interpersonal theory also had significant potential to inform the extent to which nurses could and should develop autonomous therapeutic practice, and in this sense challenged the way nurses articulated their practice across many fields. This chapter explores these debates and ideas, tracing their impact on psychiatric nursing programs and attempts to transform patient care. Going beyond psychiatric work, the ideas and practices that nurses debated reflect a critical moment in the evolution of nursing as a profession, as it sought to define the limits of nursing practice, what it meant to "care," and how that care would be valued by both patients and the psychiatric profession more broadly.

This chapter begins with an overview of the role of the NIMH in developing new graduate programs and goes on to explore the ideas that nurse leaders brought to these new programs, drawing on their writings about interpersonal relations and psychodynamic theories, and new techniques like group and milieu therapy. The postwar period was to some extent dominated by one nurse, Hildegard Peplau, and the chapter analyses her work and impact, and the debates that she engendered. Peplau represented a new generation of psychiatric nurses who took theory seriously but did not necessarily agree on what theoretical approach should inform new programs. Debates between Peplau and other nurse leaders like Dorothy Mereness and June Mellow demonstrate a lively intellectual atmosphere, which took the role of the psychiatric nurse seriously not just at the bedside but in society more broadly. Between them, these women led a generation of nurses who would take psychiatric nursing to the next level as a clinical specialty.

Toward the Teaching of Dynamic Psychiatry

The establishment of the NIMH provided new avenues for nurses in the U.S. Public Health Service to target and direct funds toward psychiatric nursing. This work was overseen initially by two highly influential women: Lucile Petry and

Esther Garrison. Petry was well established in the Public Health Service, having been the director of the Cadet Nurse Corps since 1943 and appointed as assistant surgeon general in 1949. Petry was a psychiatric nurse by training, and when the NIMH opened she recruited Garrison, her Cadet Nurse Corps mentee, to be the leader of the new Psychiatric Nursing Training and Standards Branch.[3] Encouraged by Petry and Garrison, the National League for Nursing Education (NLNE) applied for a grant to undertake a study into the quality and standards for teaching of psychiatric nursing. The survey was conducted by Mary Schmitt and published in 1949.[4] Building on Laura Fitzsimmons's earlier survey for the American Psychiatric Association (APA) and Rockefeller Foundation, Schmitt reported that in 1948 only seven university-based advanced programs existed, at Catholic University, the University of Colorado, University of Washington, University of Minnesota, University of Pittsburgh, Teachers College (TC) at Columbia University, and Boston University. All of these programs had problems with content, structure, and evaluation. Only four of them were master's programs (Colorado, TC, Minnesota, and Washington), and even here graduate students often took the same classes as undergraduate students because there were no higher-level courses offered and no one qualified to teach them. Schmitt reported that there were sixteen faculty members involved in developing and running these early programs, yet only one had a master's degree (in psychology) and three had no degrees at all. Of the sixteen, twelve had extensive clinical experience. The most pressing need the Schmitt study identified was for qualified faculty to develop and implement new curriculums.[5]

The means for the development of faculty fell largely under the purview of Garrison at the NMIH. Garrison was in charge of awarding training stipends that, supplemented by the GI Bill, provided funds for nurses to undertake graduate education at universities. She also worked with the NLNE and the American Nurses Association to organize and provide funds for conferences at which ideas and projects could be developed, and she fostered awards for pilot projects and, later, full grants for new graduate programs. Garrison had firm ideas about what form these programs should take, and she articulated these in 1953 in an article in the APA journal *Psychiatric Services*. She noted that the "movement away from teaching descriptive psychiatry to the teaching of dynamic psychiatry" and explored the emerging themes in psychiatric nursing education. Garrison described the first of these as a "major emphasis on growth and development of the personality, and on the various physical, psychological and social influences which modify this, as well as on the dynamics of behavior and of interpersonal relationships."[6] Other themes included the "growing interest in the hospital situation as a social situation," "the development of the therapeutic role of the nurse," and "the growing awareness of the nurse's role as a collaborative worker in planning and administering psychiatric care."[7] These themes drew on some of the ideas that nurses had begun to articulate before World War II; however, Garrison went further by suggesting that the basis of advanced education was in fact now heavily theoretical and actively promoted the capacity of the nurse as a therapeutic agent.

In these ideas, Garrison was reflecting debates being held across nursing leadership. Throughout the early to mid-1950s, the major nursing organizations worked together to fully articulate the functions and qualifications of the psychiatric nurse through a number of conferences, studies, and reports. In 1948 the NLNE and the National Organization for Public Health Nursing (NOPHN) formed the Joint Project in Psychiatric Nursing, which received a grant through Garrison's office at the NIMH to undertake conferences and studies aimed at setting definitive standards for practice and education. As part of this project, in 1950 the NLNE and the University of Minnesota hosted the "Conference on Advanced Psychiatric Nursing and Mental Hygiene Programs," at which a lively discussion was held about the viability of preparing nurses to "do psychotherapy." Participants agreed that "the nurse is a therapeutic force and her relationships have meaning in the treatment of patients," and that "nurses should move forward in the direction of being able to become participants in psychotherapeutic teams."[8] At the same conference a consensus was reached about the definition of psychiatric nursing, which laid out a vision for both institutional and public work: "Psychiatric nursing, as a branch of the art and science of nursing, is concerned with the total nursing care of the psychiatric patient through the development and guidance of interpersonal relationships, the creation of therapeutic situations and the application of other nursing skills used in psychiatric treatment, and with the prevention of mental illness and the promotion of mental health."[9] But this definition did not necessarily indicate the reality of psychiatric nursing work or education. It was in recognition of the disparity between the ideal and the reality that the participants at the 1950 conference also recommended to the NLNE that it form a committee to review and make recommendations on the existing guide to advanced clinical courses. The joint project sponsored two more conferences in 1951 and 1952: the 1951 conference in particular sought to clarify the functions and learning experiences for the psychiatric nursing specialist and the psychiatric nursing instructor. To further these aims, the joint project published *A Study of Desirable Functions and Qualifications for the Psychiatric Nurse*, conducted by a recent graduate from TC, Claire Mintzer Fagin.[10]

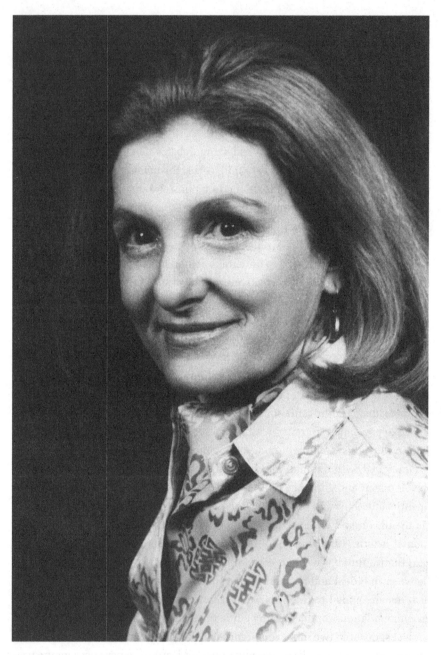

Claire M. Fagin, 1960s. Photo courtesy of the Barbara Bates Center for the Study of the History of Nursing, MC 95.

This study built on two earlier reports entitled *The Nurse Mental Health Consultant: Functions and Qualifications* and *Inventory and Qualifications for Psychiatric Nurses*. The latter, by Aurelie Nowakowski, demonstrated that while "75% of the supervisors, head nurses, and staff nurses now practicing in psychiatry have had no preparation for their position beyond their basic nursing education," it was also the case that "more than 50% of the nurses in each of these categories was interested in further study."[11] Fagin's study was designed to build on Nowakowski's and to "find out what nurses in psychiatric facilities think they are doing and what they want to do."[12] The study's findings indicated that nurses themselves saw their roles as far more expansive than had previously been imagined. Fagin and the project's Advisory Committee distilled survey responses down to six functions and seven qualifications. The functions included teaching, supervision, administration, consultation, and research, but the number-one function that nurses themselves considered desirable was "establishing relationships with people, i.e., with patients, personnel, the public, members of the 'team' etc."[13] This was especially important for the head nurse, who "establishes helpful or therapeutic relationships with patients, personnel, visitors, inter-disciplinary team members (psychologists, psychiatrists, social workers, etc.) and others."[14]

The Advisory Committee sought to expand on the definition of nursing by adding four "dynamic" functions that included collecting data related to identifying and solving problems; making inferences and judgments based on these data; acting or intervening on the basis of said inferences; and "evaluating entire processes in terms of whether problems identified have been solved."[15] These high-level conceptual skills took nursing action in psychiatry beyond tasks to a much more theoretical and abstract level, and so desirable qualifications included factors such as intelligence, attitudes, motivations; an attitude of inquiry; "trained capacity to make inferences and judgements in ways that are useful . . . in relations with patients"; warmth and empathy; imagination and resourcefulness; personal stamina, and, perhaps most importantly for this committee, "appreciations and understandings in the areas of knowledge required for psychiatric nursing."[16] In relation to this question of knowledge, the committee was careful not to limit what this should be. Rather, they recognized that the field of psychiatric theory and practice was changing so rapidly that specific delineations would not be helpful or possible. They did, however, point out that their vision of the head nurse was a person who acted as a researcher, collecting data about all aspects of patient care and outcomes, developing nursing specific activities and knowledge, and contributing to a further understanding of human nature. Therefore, they suggested that nurses engaged in research work should be "working toward a doctoral degree."[17] In this sense, Fagin's report, and the Advisory Committee attached to her project (which included Hildegard Peplau and Esther Garrison), stressed the importance of advanced knowledge through advanced education. While there was no overt agreement about what specific form this advanced education should take, the twin concepts of interpersonal relations and psychodynamic nursing were considered central.

Interpersonal Relations and Psychodynamic Nursing

The idea that the relationship between the nurse and the patient was in itself a therapeutic tool had emerged out of the rise of psychotherapy and the recognition that mental illness was often a matter of unresolved problems in relationships with others. Therefore, the nurse needed to recognize that her relationship with the patient was an integral part of their treatment. In this sense, the concept was articulated as the nurse-patient relationship and drew on already existing assumptions about this integral and personal part of nursing practice. The nature of nurse-patient relationships had been a concern of nurse leaders for some time. Their earlier calls for maturity and empathy in the psychiatric nurse had arisen from a recognition of the damaging effects that stereotypes of uncaring nurses had on attracting women to the workforce. But they also recognized that the demeanor, attitude, and beliefs of the nurse were integral to the success of patient treatment. The rise of psychotherapy pushed psychiatric nurses to engage with the nurse-patient relationship at a deeper level than they had previously, and it specifically asked them to look at themselves in this relationship.

In 1947 Helena Render published the first nurse-led book since Harriet Bailey's *Nursing Mental Diseases*. Render's text, *Nurse-Patient Relationships in Psychiatry*, explicitly referenced interpersonal relationships in an opening chapter that stressed the importance of the nurse's personality for psychiatric work.[18] Render differentiated between the nurse who was interested in "people" and the nurse who was interested in "things," suggesting that excess in either type would not be suitable to psychiatric nursing. Rather, a middle ground was necessary because Render's personality qualifications for psychiatric nursing were focused on "mastering theory and practice." The correct personality, for Render, included characteristics of "emotional maturity, adaptability, sensitive perception and discernment, creative imagination and enthusiasm, inductive reasoning or foresight, and the pioneer spirit."[19] The nurse's "principal function is to modify pathological moods and change unwholesome attitudes," and the nurse would need to work closely with both the patient and the physician in order to bring about such change.

This closeness to the patient did not mean that the nurse would or should be autonomous, however. Working at the periphery, auxiliary to the physician, Render saw psychiatric nursing as "a contributory affective therapy."[20] In a table of "Pertinent Points and Essential Concepts," Render argued that psychiatric nursing was not unique from general nursing, but that the nurse needed to "live therapy" if she was to create this successful therapeutic environment. That is, "you do not use little bits of energy now and then. You have to think continually."[21] Render went further by suggesting that the patient was in fact a teacher: in the patient's actions and reactions, "he teaches you the importance of reciprocity in human relationships and the need for honesty in social relationships. . . . The gravest lessons and the sharpest rebukes come from the patient."[22] The rapport that the nurse needed to build with the patient could not be therapeutic if the nurse was not self-aware, or open to change within herself. In this sense, Render spoke to the psychodynamic aspect of psychiatric nursing in that she emphasized the need for the nurse to study, observe, and understand the emotional underpinnings of the patient's behavior, and to notice and control those things within herself.

Yet Render's book remained largely undertheorized and vague. She referenced the same sources we saw nurses draw on in relation to mental hygiene and the function of the nurse as defined by psychiatry. There was no direct reference to psychiatric theory itself, and the emphasis was on the personal behavior and attitude of the nurse. She reminded nurses that their primary objective was to take direction from and enact the program of the physician, and provided no independent theoretical or practical framework through which the nurse could actually act therapeutically. In a retrospective review of the nursing literature related to the nurse patient relationship published in 1975, Suzanne Lego characterized Render's book and the few other articles about interpersonal relations in this immediate postwar period as problematic because "vague notions were being expressed about exactly how or in what way the psychiatric nurse could help the patient."[23] This situation, Lego argued, "abruptly ended in the literature as a result of the publication of Dr. Hildegard Peplau's book *Interpersonal Relations in Nursing* in 1952."[24]

Peplau's Idea of Nurses as Therapists

Hildegard Elizabeth Peplau was born in 1909 in Reading, Pennsylvania, to immigrant parents of German descent. Her life has been chronicled in intricate detail by her biographer, Barbara Callaway, who called her "the psychiatric nurse of the century."[25] Callaway notes that there was nothing romantic or inevitable about Peplau's path to psychiatry. While her choice of nursing was born of

practical necessity, Peplau's curiosity and interest in psychiatry was piqued by
a particular experience in her early training at Pennsylvania's Pottstown School
of Nursing—a four-day psychiatric rotation in the nearby Norristown State
Hospital. Norristown's chief psychiatrist was Dr. Arthur Noyes, who would later
go onto to be a president of the APA and someone who Peplau later recalled as
"always a helpful and clarifying spokesman for the work role of nurses in psychiatric facilities."[26] Noyes left a strong impression on Peplau. In an oral history taken in 1985, Peplau recalled that the Dr. Noyes and his staff would "bring
us in and for the first half hour or so we got a lecture on something. And then
they would bring in different kinds of schizophrenics and parade them around
the stage. And Dr Noyes would ask them to do something like hallucinate, or
tell a delusion, or show waxy flexibility. So that these peculiarities that were
described to us in the lecture were shown. . . . And then the patients would leave
and then there would be a brief discussion with Dr Noyes. And we would
regularly ask, 'Well what causes it?' . . . And he would look so sad and say 'I
honestly don't know.' We thought that was just awful."[27]

Also striking to Peplau was the community silence and stigma around
mental illness, and the conditions in which these community members now
found themselves:

> I said it was shocking and yet it wasn't shocking because all the neigh-
> borhoods that we had come from, even off the farm, had some knowl-
> edge of weird people because the tendency was to keep them at home. . . .
> The peculiarities we were seeing were not new, at least not to me. The
> others too, they saw the same things in their farm communities. . . . The
> thing that shocked me the most was that they didn't know the cause.
> The wards were clean enough, and the patients didn't look beat up.
> I was appalled by the fact that they were all lined up against the walls.
> But they weren't in shackles. They were inert.[28]

Nevertheless, Peplau did not actively pursue psychiatric nursing as a
specialty until later in her career. In 1936 she took a job at Mt. Sinai Hospital in
New York. She worked hard and made a good impression on her superiors, and
availed herself of free lectures at the New School for Social Research, where she
heard Eric Fromm and Karen Horney speak. During the summer, she worked at
the New York University (NYU) student camp as the staff nurse, and impressed
the director so much that he referred her to the director of admissions at a new
women's college in Vermont, Bennington. Encouraged by the NYU camp director and excited at the chance to be in an academic environment, she took the
job as nurse in the student health center.[29]

At Bennington she was encouraged to take classes for credit, and it was here that she encountered the new generation of psychiatric thinkers. One of her first courses was on psychology, taught by none other than Eric Fromm himself.[30] By the 1940s, the college was home to some of the most influential names in psychology and psychiatry, with luminaries like Fromm, Frieda Fromm-Reichmann, and Harry Stack Sullivan all contributing to the program. Peplau's reading list and her extensive lecture notes reveal a challenging, confronting, and stimulating program of study covering topics from aggression and frustration, basic personality structure, psychoanalysis, hypnosis, dream interpretation, and interpersonal relations.[31] Peplau also undertook clinical placements at Chestnut Lodge in Rockville, Maryland, where she attended weekly seminars and discussion groups with Sullivan. At Chestnut Lodge she worked intensively with Fromm-Reichmann, who believed psychoanalysis had a significant role to play in the treatment of schizophrenia and taught Peplau the principles of one-to-one therapy.

When America entered World War II in 1941, Peplau was keen to apply what she had learned at Bennington and rushed to complete her final year of study so she could enlist in the U.S. Army Nurse Corps.[32] She was eventually shipped to the 3-12th Field Station and School for Military Neuropsychiatry in the south of England in late 1943. Established by William Menninger as the psychiatric consultant to the U.S. Army surgeon general, and formed in collaboration with some of the United Kingdom's best-known practitioners from the Tavistock Clinic, the 3-12th considered itself at the cutting edge of military neuropsychiatry.[33] For all its talk about innovation, however, the therapeutic approach at the 3-12th was at best ambiguous. As a school, it was responsible for the very rapid training (or upskilling) of military medical officers into make-shift psychiatrists, and drew on consultant psychologists, psychiatrists, army medics, and career military nurses to effect treatment as quickly as possible.[34] That treatment was almost always experimental, and primarily designed to get soldiers back on the battlefield as soon as possible. Psychiatry was in the man-power business during the war, and this agenda allowed a space where experimentation with no informed consent and no scientific evidence was the norm. These therapies included subsequently discredited treatments such as insulin shock and deep sleep therapy, and the use of drug-induced abreaction, which Peplau found particularly distasteful.[35]

She was disturbed by the program of treatment at the 3-12th for a number of reasons. It was often inhumanely administered, based on restraint and physical and psychological violence, and employed by unskilled medics or attendants who preferred these methods because they reinforced army notions of hierarchy and control. In 1944 she explained this dilemma to her sister: "I've contributed heavily towards indoctrinating toward the humane method—the other way is easier and for some reason appeals to medics. It was a crushing blow to me to learn the discrepancy between office and army practice, between ideal and actual treatments."[36] Peplau agitated her superiors for the chance to try something different and was eventually given charge of a ward where she established an occupational and group therapy program that impressed her supervisor, Jay Hoffman.[37]

After the war, with the support of the GI Bill, Peplau enrolled in the master's program at TC, but she was frustrated by the level of instruction. In an oral history she recalled that "the person in charge of the program was Carolyn Fowles, and she was from the Community Services Society and she was not a psychiatric nurse. . . . She tried, and she brought in various people to give lectures. And they would tell us how good or bad their golf games were."[38] Importantly, one person who did make a favorable impression on Peplau was Laura Fitzsimmons. "She was remarkable," Peplau recalled. "I learned a great deal from her about the overall picture of psychiatric nursing. In fact, when push comes to shove, she's about the only one I care to remember. I was livid. And then when they had us cutting up paper napkins to make doilies in case we ever had to entertain patients I hit the ceiling. I really went into a rage . . . so they wrote into my record that I was emotionally disturbed. Probably not recommendable for any job."[39] Nevertheless Peplau graduated in 1947 and went on to undertake several important clinical roles outside New York City.

It soon became obvious to some that Peplau was a rising star in the field: Esther Garrison at the NIMH was particularly proactive in earmarking certain people for support and money, and Peplau had not escaped her attention.[40] The new dean of nursing at TC, Louise McManus, was keen to have Peplau return, which she finally did in September 1948.[41] The irony of her return to TC was not lost on Peplau. "Having made such a big stink about how bad it was, I have now the onus of making it better," she recalled. "And there were absolutely no guidelines. Everything that was published up until then was absolutely worthless, with one or two exceptions. The psychiatric nursing textbooks were watered down descriptive psychiatry."[42] Peplau tried to think of new ways of approaching teaching that would work toward building autonomous practice for the nurse. She recalled the lessons she had learned from Frieda Fromm-Reichmann at Chestnut Lodge, and through her own personal psychoanalysis at the William Alanson White Institute. Through these experiences, she worked on refining her theory about what constituted both nursing practice and a method for nurse education. This work was designed to articulate a clear body of nursing

knowledge—nursing expertise developed by and for nurses that would facilitate the development of advanced practice in psychiatric nursing. Specifically,
this was knowledge of psychoanalytic and psychotherapeutic theory, which she
combined with Sullivan's practical work on interpersonal relations to spell out
a very distinct role for the nurse. She called this role psychodynamic nursing,
the model for which she eventually published in the text *Interpersonal Relations in Nursing: A Conceptual Frame of Reference for Psychodynamic
Nursing.*[43]

At TC Peplau created an innovative and exciting learning environment.
Fagin recalled the exhilaration and inspiration of that time, the feeling that the
students were part of something new and special:

> Methods I learned there were learned because there were people who
> were so extraordinary. . . . Hilda had a way of teaching that would make
> you feel that you had to rush to the library immediately because she threw
> things around in class, not in the way that was confusing but in a way
> that was stimulating, so intellectually seducing, if you will, that all you
> wanted to do was run out of that class and run like some crazy person to
> the library to look up all these things. She never told you to do it, it was
> never said to you, it was the way she taught. You saw this intellectual
> work, the way she used names, the way she used their theories you had
> to know more. Now I never had an experience like that. Now, that was
> extraordinary.[44]

Despite this environment (or perhaps because of it), personal conflicts at
TC made Peplau restless, and when she was approached by Ella Stonsby to
establish a program at Rutgers University in New Jersey, she expressed interest.
She did not accept, however, until she was sure she would be able to run the
program the way she wanted, including the ability to organize intensive clinical placements for her students. Once this plan was in place, Peplau applied
to the NIMH for funding and was awarded a grant for the program at Rutgers
in 1954.[45]

In her oral history, Peplau recalled the environment in which nurses sought
to create programs at this time: "Our task was to create advanced psychiatric
nursing practice, because there was no such thing. . . . And we were working in
isolation. . . . We were all burdened with all sorts of things to get our programs
started, to get the content developed, to get the field work going, admit the students, deal with the students' problems. It was just tremendous."[46] At Rutgers
the essence of Peplau's program was psychotherapy. Students themselves under-
went analysis and this self-development was combined with theory and clinical

case studies. She arranged placements for students at Greystone Park Psychiatric Hospital and students spent intensive time there with a patient, talking and
recording observations. This was a practice that Peplau had learned from
Fromm-Reichmann: listening to even the most delusional and schizophrenic
patients could reveal meaning and symbols in their "word salad." At Rutgers
she was able to fully realize her vision of training students as therapists: "They
were moving in the direction of psychotherapy. . . . We didn't call it that, we
called it 1:1 and we called it 'Talking with Patients', and then we called it
counselling and then we called it therapy. That took from 1948 until 1960."[47]

"Talking with patients" was the essence of Peplau's therapeutic approach.
She set out in *Interpersonal Relations in Nursing*, her subsequent text *Basic
Principles of Patient Counseling*, and many other articles[48] the techniques and
strategies for nurse-directed therapy that were part of whole patient care. This
method "requires a marked shift in emphasis from telling a patient how to
behave in line with preconceived goals of the nurse, toward helping the patient
to inquire and to find out what is going on with him."[49] It also required the active
presence of the nurse, that she know her own values and anxieties, and that she
put aside her judgments and need to control and learn to listen. This way of
working was in direct contrast to the paternalism inherent to existing theories
of care, which saw the nurses' role as to do for the patient what they were unable
to do for themselves. Shifting the focus to the patient required the nurse to resist
her urge to fix and control, and demanded instead that she facilitate the patient's
own experience. This was a major refocusing of the goal of nursing practice, and
was made possible through the framework of psychodynamic nursing.

Psychodynamic nursing was psychodynamic because it was an active therapeutic practice, requiring the active involvement of the nurse in both her own,
and her patient's, development. For nurses this meant self-awareness, maturity,
critical thinking, emotional openness, and reflection. But it also meant an active
engagement with psychiatric and psychological theory. Hence, the psychodynamic role of the nurse in treatment and care was predicated on a particular
theoretical understanding of what constituted mental illness. Nurses needed to
understand this theory before they could hope to be effective practitioners. Psychodynamic practitioners believed that mental health and illness occurred on
a scale, contrary to the abrupt-onset disease model. There were only gradations
between health and illness, which were exacerbated by relationships with other
people and living situations.[50] Peplau argued that the hospital setting was useful in this regard. "Helping patients to learn about the patterns of living they
use regularly, in the ward situation, by means of experiential teaching"[51] was a
key part of the nurse's role. To facilitate this learning, it was essential that nurses

were fully trained in therapeutic skills that went beyond "traditional" nursing practices such as socializing and diversion. "There are . . . still many nurses in psychiatry," she argued, "who feel that kindness, sympathy, homelike surrounding, and a little discipline is all that patients need. I do not mean to disparage these efforts. But . . . the nurse has the additional task of assisting the patient to struggle with the problem and to learn something from this experience with a nurse."[52]

The role of the nurse for Peplau was not just to understand what the psychiatrist was thinking or doing so as to complement "his" approach, but to be able to develop autonomous and active therapeutic nursing practice. This idea rested on the obvious fact that it was the nurse who was in the best position to provide the most intensive care. Peplau made this point in a presentation to the Veterans Administration Hospital in Roanoke, Virginia, in 1954, in which she argued that even when a patient was in a state of panic or sedated, the nurse had a special role to play that the physician could (and would) not, and this was simply "to be with" the patient. "It seems to me that the patient gains ground in the direction of health when someone is available to sit out these experiences with disturbed patients. And in the process of sitting it out, a nurse can provide thereness, a tangible focus, and at the same time aid the patient to struggle with the problem at hand."[53] This was not simply a passive "being with," however.

Rather, the key to Peplau's work was the translation of complex psychoanalytic and psychodynamic theories and concepts into a model for nursing action. That is, Peplau did not just tell nurses what they needed to know about human psychology, or that they should just listen and talk to patients. She also demonstrated how the theory of interpersonal relations translated into actual therapeutic action and provided tools with which the nurse could guide these interactions toward a stated goal. She did this by articulating the phases of the nurse-patient relationship, which progressed from "Orientation" to "Identification/Exploitation" and then to "Resolution." Within these phases the nursing role moved from Stranger, to Unconditional Mother Surrogate, to Counselor/Resource Person/Leadership Surrogate, to Adult Person. At the same time, the patient role changed from Stranger, to Infant, to Child, to Adolescent, to Adult person.

This twin growth trajectory meant that the nurse and patient started on equal footing, and needed to grow together toward the Adult role, in which interpersonal conflicts had been resolved. Peplau explained the intellectual tasks of the nurse within each phase. These required an unpacking of the influences that generated particular situations that the nurse may encounter and depended on expanding the "psychological tasks" with which the nurse and patient should be involved. In other words, nurses needed to be prepared to engage in meaningful discussion that led to an understanding of the patient and their circumstances and environment, and she needed to know complex theories of personality and social development. The reliance on theory meant that nurses would be able to approach each patient with a grounding in knowledge of human development and be able to identify the moments where her patient had been influenced one way or another, and then to be able to reinfluence the patient toward "adulthood." It was only with this grounding in theory that nurses would be able to understand their patients as people requiring empathy and understanding rather than judgment and fear.[54] Within *Interpersonal Relations*, Peplau set out techniques for guided discussion, and theoretical explanations for fear, anxiety, and withdrawal. She provided extensive case studies and detailed explanations of how to interpret particular phrases and how to respond without causing more harm. The book was a masterful intertwining of ideas from Sullivan, Freud, Horney, and Fromm-Reichmann, and took the theoretical underpinnings of psychiatric nursing to a new level. Most importantly, it provided a clear rationale and program for nurses to act as autonomous therapeutic agents.

Mereness and the Push for Autonomous Practice

The idea that nurses were in a unique position to contribute to therapeutic outcomes was also taken up by another psychiatric nurse, Dorothy Mereness. Away from the intellectual hotbed of New York City, Mereness found herself dealing with many of the same issues that troubled Peplau. She had left teaching for nursing in 1938, studying at Case Western Reserve. In her third year there, she took a class on psychiatric nursing and realized this was what she had been looking for, a way to understand and articulate the complexities of human behavior.[55] The class was directed by Professor Louis L. Karnosh, author of *Psychiatry for Nurses* (1940), one of only two texts concerned with psychiatric nursing at that time (the other being Harriet Bailey's *Nursing Mental Diseases*). Karnosh was also director of the Psychiatric Division of Cleveland Hospital, and it was at his recommendation that Mereness was offered a job as an instructor of psychiatric nursing at City Hospital in Cleveland. She became coauthor of subsequent editions of Karnosh's text, and eventually the sole author of the well-respected and highly utilized *Essentials of Psychiatric Nursing*.

Karnosh was a significant influence on Mereness in both her approach to nursing practice and her career progression. In her memories of Karnosh, she discusses the influence of psychoanalysis on their work together and also the issues that faced psychiatric theory outside the urban centers, explaining that Karnosh was often forced to deny Freud because of the sexual focus of the latter's work: "I think it was because Freud said a lot about sex that it was considered to be a bad thing. Everyone admired Dr. Karnosh a lot; he was a married man with three children, an outstanding citizen, so he couldn't possibly believe in Freud."[56] Mereness's insistence on the creation of knowledge for autonomous practice stemmed from her early work at City Hospital, and later at the University of Pittsburgh, where she undertook her graduate psychiatric nurse training. At City Hospital Mereness struggled to introduce more humane therapeutic methods in the face of continual practices of restraint: "I'd go up on the unit—they were always putting people in straitjackets—and I'd take them out."[57] At the University of Pittsburgh in 1947, theory was everything, but it was not nursing theory. She read psychiatric journals and recognized how little she knew, despite her extensive clinical and practical experience. As she discovered, clinical experience was considered nothing without a theoretical framework with which to analyze both patient behavior and approaches to treatment and care.[58] This is a significant point, because nurses at this time had so little exposure to psychiatric theory that the main source of nursing knowledge *was* experience.

This issue was a constant source of tension in Mereness's work. She attempted to balance the knowledge of experience with the knowledge of emerging theory, and to turn that theory into something of practical use to nurses. She did so for the first time as part of her studies at the University of Pittsburgh, where she saw an opening for developing nursing practice as part of the mental health team:

> One of the things we used to do at Pitt—we used to sit around a table to discuss a patient. That is, the psychologists, social workers, psychiatrists sat around the table. The nurses would sit around the wall. And sometimes they knew more about the patient than anybody. And I would sometimes say "Miss So-and So knows a good deal about the patient. If you would drag her out and demand that she talk she could tell you a great deal." We tried to get nurses who knew the patient to sit at the table. We had a terrible time getting them to sit at the table.[59]

Her experiences led her to write her first journal article, "Preparation of the Nurse for the Psychiatric Team," which was published in 1951.[60] In it she stressed the importance of an academic and intellectual background that would give nurses both the knowledge and the confidence to be taken seriously within the team, as well as have her extensive practical and clinical experience recognized. The nurse must have a thorough grounding in theory, be able to communicate clearly, be reflective, and be capable of working in a team.[61] In an oral history she recalled the lack of teamwork at City Hospital and how this article, so central to her thinking, was used in an attempt to challenge that. "They had my paper reproduced and put on all the doctors' desks . . . and I did my doctorate on that, I went up to NYU and set up a graduate program based on that, based on the fact that the nurse had to be as well prepared theoretically as the physician. That they have to be respected, to be knowledgeable."[62] This was a central tenet of both Peplau's and Mereness's visions: that nurses needed to know theoretically why they should act in a certain way, so that they could challenge or complement the psychiatrist as appropriate. It was also essential if nurses were going to be mindful, aware and therapeutic agents in their own right, and no longer dismissed as merely handmaidens or attendants.

In her 1951 article, Mereness also explicitly referred to the concept of inter-personal relations and its significance for team members.[63] By now, Peplau was making her presence felt beyond New York City. She had given a workshop at the University of Pittsburgh that Mereness had attended, and her presence had left stars in many students' eyes: "I heard some people talking about someone as if she were a superhuman, a marvelous person, and then I realized they were talking about Miss Peplau, and then I thought if there's this person who knows so much, I must involve myself with her."[64] Mereness's desire for formal quali-fications and thirst for new knowledge sent her to TC in New York to undertake her PhD. By the time she had applied and been accepted to the program at TC, however, Peplau had already left. Mereness was frustrated but undeterred: "When I went there it was to study with her. I was so distressed and went to talk with her." She nevertheless resolved to stay at TC and get what she could out of a program she felt was lesser for the absence of Peplau.[65] While Mereness had initially hoped to undertake a PhD, the nature of the program at TC (aimed at producing nurse educators, not clinical specialists), meant that she was even-tually awarded an EdD in 1956.

Soon after Mereness started at TC, she met Martha Rogers, dean of nursing at NYU. Rogers recruited Mereness to the faculty of NYU while she was still completing her doctorate at TC, and then added her name to an application to the NIMH for an advanced practice program in psychiatric nursing for the col-lege. Mereness was given control of setting up that program.[66] Many of the major nursing schools in U.S. universities were keen to take advantage of the funds offered by the NIMH, and Mereness noted the varying effects this had on the development of curriculums. "Different places were developing different ideas. . . . We all got similar amounts of money, and all had to beat the bushes for their first class."[67] When NYU set up its program, she recalled that "people were horrified that they'd given a grant to run in competition with TC. I think NIMH wanted someone to run in competition with TC. There was never any relationship at all [between TC, NYU, and Rutgers]. They never met together, never talked together. They were all too competitive for students."[68]

Mereness was well aware of the shadow cast at the time by Peplau, whom she remembered as "the leading person in psychiatry" considered "the king of all she surveyed."[69] Peplau's shadow was indeed long, but Mereness had her own ideas about what the program at NYU should look like. For her, the emphasis of nursing practice in mental health should be on the family, and this seemed to put her at odds with Peplau: "I always started my students out in nursery schools. Miss Peplau didn't agree with that at all. . . . She said once, although she never told me, that she thought this was a terrible waste of time."[70] Mereness's conception of mental illness was always grounded in the family, and she believed that nurses themselves had long understood this, observing that "the patient is forced to utilize a psychotic reaction as the possible defense available in light of the situation and his family's response."[71] However, in order to be able to deal with such volatile family situations, nurses needed a firm grounding in theory. As she developed her program at NYU, Mereness drew on the language of interpersonal relations and argued that the nurse had a unique opportunity to provide therapeutic care through the use of psychodynamic and interpersonal nursing. She argued that this would not be possible, however, if nurses did not know the theory behind this type of practice, and without it they were of no benefit to patients. The nurse, she insisted, "needs a good understanding of the use of psychological principles to apply to nursing care; a knowledge of psychodynamic theory in order to understand the behavior of patients and her interactions with them."[72]

Importantly, however, Mereness recognized the difficulty nurses would face in implementing psychodynamic nursing in existing institutional systems. The prevailing philosophy of the psychiatrist in charge within most inpatient facilities would necessarily limit or alter the kind of work that nurses could do. "Medical philosophy and psychiatric treatment programs alter the role of the nurse in a profound and direct way,"[73] she acknowledged. In this sense, her ideas about the role of nurses within institutions were arguably more practical in nature than Peplau's. Whereas Peplau had decried the "socializing" or diversionary nature of some nursing work in inpatient facilities, Mereness thought this was valuable work in relation to providing a safe space for patients. In this thinking, she drew explicitly on theories of milieu therapy, and advocated that nurses should be familiar with this theory in order to provide the most conducive environment, regardless of the institutional approach.[74]

These differences in theoretical and practical approaches to the development of educational programs were not seen as problematic at the time. In the absence of any pre-existing advanced-practice programs, each program was able to address itself to what its leaders saw as specific needs within the psychiatric nursing workforce. For Mereness, the emphasis was on developing a new generation of nurses who could take the profession through the challenges to come, carving out a space not just for nursing at the psychiatric bedside but also at the policy table. In 1985 she recalled, "Miss Peplau saw the role of the psychiatric nurse as a therapist, and she should have the credit for developing the role of therapist. . . . We had the concept at NYU of preparing leaders. . . . We thought they ought to know a great deal about patients, about patient behavior, and patient care, but we thought they would be directing other people. . . . I think direct care is a very limited kind of influence."[75] For Mereness, it was not just that nurses needed clinical knowledge to be able to hold their own in clinical practice. They also needed to be able to take control of their own profession, which required knowledge, skill, and confidence. Mereness saw this gap in nurse education and used her position at NYU, and later as dean of the School of Nursing at the University of Pennsylvania, to continually advocate for nurses to take charge of their own place in the psychiatric mental health team, and within the profession more broadly. Advanced education was essential to this process.

In a speech to nurses at Montrose Veterans Hospital in New York, Mereness stressed the need for more nurses working in psychiatry to undertake advanced degrees. Without this, nursing would struggle to be taken seriously as a profession, and nurses would not be able to develop their own approach to practice. "Part of the difficulty," Mereness argued, "arises from the fact that some nurses who are currently practicing have a limited understanding of psychodynamic theory. Without a reliable theoretical base it is almost impossible to develop therapeutic practices which are predicated upon more than intuitive guesses."[76] In this she drew directly from Peplau, arguing that while a therapeutic use of self and a commitment to emotional connection was required of nurses, it was still paramount that these be supported by a knowledge of theory, and that this theoretical knowledge be used to "develop research programs that could contribute data to the understanding of human behavior."[77] As with most theories, however, the true test was in the application, and in how it responded to real-world situations.

Applying Peplau's Theory

Some nurses were quick to adapt the theory of interpersonal relations as Peplau had developed it into research and interventions. Group therapy, family therapy, and milieu therapy were also emerging in the psychiatric field at this time, and were employed eagerly by the first generation of graduates from the programs established by women like Peplau and Mereness. Their work showed the impact that the theory of interpersonal relations had on mental health nursing knowledge and the different ways in which it could now be applied to nursing practice and research. Peplau's first cohorts at TC included women such as Claire Fagin, Gwen Tudor, and Ildaura Murillo-Rohde. We have already seen Fagin's impact through her work with the NLNE/NOPHN Joint Project and the articulation of functions and qualifications for psychiatric nursing as a clinical specialty. Fagin would go on to have an even greater impact in her work on child psychiatry, but it was Tudor who initially took up Peplau's call for research in interpersonal relations.

In a study entitled "A Sociopsychiatric Nursing Approach to Intervention in a Problem of Mutual Withdrawal on a Mental Hospital Ward," Tudor actively sought to demonstrate the processes of interpersonal relations and evaluate their effectiveness when deployed by a nurse in a ward setting.[78] The study took a further step by connecting interpersonal theory with sociological theory, arguing that the relationships between the nurse and the patient needed to be understood in the context of the total environment. Tudor herself was the investigator and the study took place at Chestnut Lodge under the supervision of Dr. Morris Schwartz, the facility's research sociologist.[79] In the introduction to the study, Tudor wrote, "Psychiatric nurses in a mental hospital are increasingly expected to manifest their competence in nursing by an awareness of and an ability to handle their interpersonal relations with patients in a therapeutically useful manner."[80] The nurses' activities would, in this scenario, manifest in three specific directions: facilitating the patients communications, facilitating the patients social participation, and helping to fulfil the patient's needs. To do this effectively, the nurse needed to understand the social context of the hospital ward, which was necessarily constraining and itself constitutive of patient behavior. The nurse also needed to understand herself as part of this social context, as constrained and affected by and maintaining of it. If mental illness was to be understood as an interpersonal problem, or a problem in living, then the road to recovery "can be altered and influenced by the activities others direct towards [the patient]" within the hospital setting, and this was a process for which the nurse needed to be responsible.[81] Tudor's study design echoed parts of the NLNE definition of psychiatric nursing (the process of drawing inferences through observation and designing interventions based on that data), when she elaborated an iterative process of observation, evaluation, intervention, re-evaluation, and further intervention as the basis for nursing processes. Her goal then was to determine to what extent this iterative process helped to "alter modes of social participation in the direction of increased security, satisfaction, and higher self-esteem for the patient."[82] As she reported on the developing relationship between the nurse and patients, she observed the effect of the nurses' attitudes and behavior on the tendency of the patient to withdraw or not, and at the same time she had discussions with the nursing and aide staff about their behavior, attitudes, activities, and language that were possibly impacting their relationship with patients.

The study found that the nurse-patient relationship evolved through various phases toward a more mature or adult type of relationship where animosity or mistrust was eventually reduced, much as Peplau had laid out in her book.[83] It also found that the more the nurse withdrew from a therapeutic relationship, the more the patient withdrew from the treatment process. The significance of this finding for Tudor was that in her role as the investigator she could actively observe and intervene in these situations, and explain the process to other nurses as she did so, so that "the process of mutual withdrawal was interrupted and significant alterations in the patient's mode of participation occurred."[84] While the study was not extensive enough to determine whether this favorable change followed through to an eventual cure of the patient, Tudor felt justified in concluding that "psychotherapy—the intensive investigation of the patients difficulties in living—must be integrated and coordinated with sociopsychiatric nursing care in order to consolidate and continue the improvement."[85]

Tudor's study identified the ways in which psychiatric nurses could apply the theory of interpersonal relations and theories from other disciplines to develop new directions in research and practice. The study was also groundbreaking in that it gave nurses new ways of conceptualizing the social system of institutions, which moved nursing practice away from tasks to therapy, but also moved nursing research into the realm of social science. Gwen Tudor Will (her married name) went on to design the psychiatric nursing program at the National Institutes of Health's first mental health Clinical Center when it opened in 1953 and subsequently became the chief of psychiatric nursing there.[86] In this role, she acted as a consultant (along with Kathleen Black and others) to the Group for the Advancement of Psychiatry in the production of its 1955 report *Therapeutic Use of The Self: A Concept for Teaching Patient Care*.[87] In this report, professional psychiatry's attitude toward nursing practice was informed by knowledge that nurses had themselves developed, and not the other way around.

This did not mean that nurses were suddenly accepted as therapists or that institutional practices were transformed. In her historical review of the concept of group therapy, Helen Nakagawa writes that nursing texts were written in such a way as to downplay the therapeutic role of the nurse. "The imputation," she remarks, "was that nurses were not skilled enough to be doing psychotherapy. They merely happened to be therapeutic by chance. In reality, this theme was a cover to allay the anxieties of other disciplines who somehow were seen to have prerogatives over therapeutic activities. The sadness is that, for so long, not only did the other disciplines believe this, so did nurses. It was not until the early 1960s that nursing texts and articles dropped the pretense that nurses do not perform psychotherapy and began to freely use the term."[88] It had been this tension that had necessitated Peplau's obfuscation about her teaching goals and techniques in order not to upset the fragile egos of psychiatrists and superintendents. Yet the inclusion of psychodynamic theory and techniques did not necessarily free new nursing knowledge from some of its earlier tensions; nor did it translate immediately into transformed patient care.

Competing Ideas about Care and Control

New graduate courses produced such small numbers of students that the idea of nurses as therapists did not readily translate to improvements in patient care. If the insistence on theory, therapy, and interpersonal relations revealed anything, it was the continued reality of life and practice in the psychiatric hospital. The 1950s saw an increase in psychiatric hospitalization, with no commensurate increase in staffing numbers. Conditions in public hospitals in particular were well known to be merely custodial, with active care minimal at best, and violence against patients all too frequent. Nurses were not helpless in the face of these issues, however: they could and did speak out. A classmate of Fagin and Tudor's, Ildaura Murillo-Rohde, used the knowledge she had gained in her classes with Peplau to transform institutional practice when she became assistant superintendent of nursing at Wayne County Psychiatric Hospital, Michigan, in 1954. She recalled the state of the hospital when she arrived: "4500 patients and 1500 employees, most were psychiatric attendants, and few RNs or LPNs." Many patients were in restraints, which included the "Muff," a leather tube which encased the patients hands and attached to the wrists with a tight metal buckle. "One patient had lost one hand in the 'Muff' because of poor care."[89] Murillo-Rohde directly ordered Thorazine from the manufacturers and had it distributed to patients with the approval of the supervising psychiatrists. She then instituted better training of the attendant and nursing staff, required a list of patients in restraints delivered to her desk every day, complete with explanations for the use of restraints. This reduced the total number of patients in restraints from 360 to only six within three months. She filled fifteen registered nurse vacancies and applied for money for more, and hired a bachelor's-prepared registered nurse whom she trained in "group process to work with patients, from unit to unit." The rise in morale of both patients and staff was noticed by the medical superintendent, who had her institute the same processes at the general hospital.[90]

While Murillo-Rohde saw the usefulness in pharmaceuticals in this facility, they were not always met with approval, and most nurses trained in interpersonal relations were opposed to institutional somatic practices like pharmaceutical prescription or electroconvulsive therapy (ECT). Fagin recalled that the use of drugs and other somatic treatments was seen as a necessary evil, to be got out of the way so that the real therapeutic work could be done.[91] Peplau herself was repeatedly outspoken about the use of somatic treatments, arguing that if the nurse was given a chance to talk with the patient before other treatments were administered then the patient could be made calm and less damage would be done.

Peplau remembered a particular confrontation with a psychiatrist at a conference that epitomized her point of view and the opposition that nurses faced:

> At this conference my paper followed that of Dr. Kalinoski. So before reading it, I took a few moments to comment on the evils of EST [electroshock therapy] and that I was encouraging nurses who found EST abhorrent to not participate—taking care of patients afterwards, of course, helping them to get reoriented. But that nurses time could better be spent helping patients get oriented without EST while their faculties were still intact. Dr. K was extremely upset—agitated—as he said "at the audacity of a nurse criticizing an MD what did nurses know?" Dr. Stainbrook the chairman defended the right of everyone present to have and to express an opinion. Needless to say I wasn't too popular later at the meeting.[92]

The tensions in ideas about treatment and care were not always a simple opposition between nurses and psychiatrists. Indeed, not all nurses accepted that theoretical psychotherapy was the only or required framework through which to conceptualize nursing work. For example, from the mid-1950s June Mellow began publishing her work on nursing therapy, which she had been developing through a Public Health Service grant to the Massachusetts Mental Health Center. Mellow argued that the task of the nurse therapist, especially for a patient in the acute phase, was to make a connection with the patient that would help restore emotional equilibrium.[93] Mellow and her team published a number of articles based on their work with schizophrenic patients, and she articulated a model that relied on the establishment of loving relationships with patients and sought to undo some of the damage that had been done through previously dysfunctional interpersonal relationships.[94] While Mellow used the term "interpersonal relations," and referred to the nurse-patient relationship and one-to-one relationships, her work was not heavily theoretical in the same way that Peplau's was. Rather, she stressed the role of simple communication, which was often nonverbal, and the importance of the nurse "being there" with the patient. While she warned against many of the same transference and "rescue phantasy" issues that Peplau sought to correct by sending her own students to therapy, Mellow did not advocate for that therapy. Rather she argued that nurses needed to be able to make an emotional commitment to patients regardless of their own fears and anxieties, and to "help the patient with his overwhelming and conflicting feelings of love and hate towards her."[95]

In the same way that Peplau had articulated phases of the nurse-patient relationship, so did Mellow, but the latter articulated them in practical terms that would already be familiar to the practicing nurse. That is, Mellow's first phase involved establishing contact and building a relationship; the second phase "consists of handling the problems in the relationship once it has been established," and the third, or terminal phase, "consists of dealing with dependency feelings and separation anxieties."[96] In her articulation of how the nurse was to behave in each of these phases, Mellow used language fairly familiar to the educated psychiatric nurse in that she saw the role of the nurse as actively therapeutic through deliberate personal connection rather than the "doing for" of basic nursing tasks.[97] And while she stressed the importance of "certain personal qualifications" such as attitude and personality type, she tended to characterize these as inherent traits rather than learned skills. There is no doubt that Mellow's work articulated a way of being with patients that sought to use the therapeutic potential of the nurse in a more deliberate fashion, but her ideas did not seek to make the leap to active psychotherapy that Peplau's did.

This difference between Mellow and Peplau was the subject of a debate held at Yale later in their careers, in which Mellow argued that she felt therapeutic psychiatric work was artistic rather than scientific and that it was more natural for women as it relied on their allegedly natural capacity for love and empathy. Other nurses at the symposium tended to agree with her, as this conception seemed to be about caring, which is what nursing really was, surely? Peplau argued that her approach was also caring, but more concerned with the "enduring nature of the results"; that is, it was more scientific and evidence-based. She argued for the ability to approach psychiatric work in such a fashion that reliable results could be predicted, and that this would then also contribute to knowledge about mental illness itself. She insisted that "there are scientific aspects to [psychiatric nursing] that we can develop—that there are reliable explanatory theories in this field as there are in other fields."[98]

Mellow had raised an interesting point about gender in interpersonal relations, however. In a way she reflected arguments that earlier psychiatrists had made about the essentially caring and gentle nature of women that was in and of itself therapeutic. These gendered stereotypes seemed to spill over into the nursing scholarship. None of the literature about psychodynamic nursing in the 1950s was written by men. Journal articles published by men throughout the 1950s focused almost entirely on the education of the aide, or the scientific or technical aspects of somatic treatments such as ECT. This despite the fact that a male training school had existed in Philadelphia since 1915 (the Pennsylvania Hospital School of Nursing for Men). One of its graduates, Luther Christman, would go on to have significant influence in nursing in the late 1960s, but was actively shunned by psychiatric nursing prior to then.[99] Mellow's comment reflected the reality of the psychiatric nursing workforce in which gender had always played, and continued to play, a complicating role. Once the terrain for psychiatric work began to shift away from the institution to the community, this divide continued to widen and the framework of interpersonal relations was adapted to the new fields of family and community nursing, which remained the purview of women.

Toward Family and Community Nursing

By the late 1950s and early 1960s, psychiatric nursing was well aware of the downsizing of institutions in favor of community-based mental health services. Nurses were very quick to shift their attention to this new arena. This is hardly surprising—the emphasis on one-to-one patient relationships and the idea of the nurse as a therapist was hard to replicate in the reality of overcrowded and underfunded large-scale public institutions. Small private hospitals were more conducive to this kind of work, and more amenable to nurse-led therapy, but the opportunity to be truly autonomous most clearly presented itself in community-based outpatient clinic settings.

Mereness in particular was intently aware of the opportunities and challenges the shift from institutions to communities presented for both nursing knowledge and the profession as a whole. She saw in this space an opportunity for nurses to redefine their practice and become meaningful members of the community health team, providing a new and innovative service. Not only did this form of care create a new space for nursing, it also provided potential benefits for patients. In contrast to large impersonal institutions, "the day-care center represents a safe, rational, and consistent environment which provides a maximum opportunity for interpersonal interaction with both staff and other patients."[100]

Sensing the very real changes that deinstitutionalization would have on both patients and the profession, Mereness argued that the current model of public health nursing was inadequate and that "this area may be the most fruitful one in which to expand the role of the psychiatric nurse to provide an opportunity for her to make a unique contribution to community mental health."[101] In the same way that nurses had once argued for the inclusion of mental hygiene in public health work, Mereness now argued for psychiatric nurses to be involved in the emerging community mental health movement. The rapidly evolving nature of the profession meant that nurses needed to be ready to step outside traditional roles and accept the new challenges presented by the move to community-based services, whatever form they might take. Mereness argued that "the psychiatric nurse is one of the key professional workers in such a situation and greatly influences the environment through which the decisions are made and the information which is communicated."[102] It was in this context that she articulated her vision for a nurse-led community health team. Nurses had special skills that enabled effective community health work, and they should, she argued, be "working toward developing and transforming the role in order to bring into reality the concept of a psychiatric nurse-psychiatrist team."[103] In this scenario, the psychiatric nurse would develop and lead the treatment plan in consultation with the rest of the team.

But the great benefit of the move toward community-based services, for Mereness, was the opportunity for nurses to work more closely with families.[104] The nurse who was trained in family therapy had a significant role to play in new community settings because she could situate the patient in their family and social environment, and in this space she could be instrumental in helping to "re-establish meaningful communication between the disturbed individual and his human environment,"[105] thus assisting not just the person, but the whole family to move on from pathological forms of behavior. Working with families and children through a model of interpersonal relations proved particularly attractive to mental health nurses. Building on the history of public health and visiting nursing, it seemed to fit so naturally with the work they had always done with families and children, and gave new frameworks, and new legitimacy, to the development of autonomous work.

Nurses such as Grayce Sills, Shirley Smoyak, and Claire Fagin opened up new terrain in this space through their engagement with interpersonal relations.

They applied that theory and theories from the social sciences to their work with groups and families to create new ways of thinking about the nursing role and the nurse-patient relationship. As a student and then colleague of Peplau's at Rutgers, Smoyak recalled the way in which systems theory was incorporated into the conceptual framework so as to bring deeper understanding of the role of the family in mental illness, and to facilitate working with the patient as a product of their whole environment.[106] Smoyak herself completed her PhD in sociology at Rutgers and went on to be a professor and run the university's graduate program. She continued to publish extensively on the idea of the nurse as family therapist, as did Mereness herself. Fagin, who had been working at the Clinical Center in Bethesda, Maryland, was encouraged by Mereness to contact her if she ever returned to New York, and when she did, Mereness employed her to develop the new graduate program at NYU. It was when Fagin was working at NYU that her own son was taken ill and she argued with nursing staff about leaving him alone because of hospital visiting rules. The nurses accused her of building an unhealthy dependency, and Fagin, well-versed in the theories developed by Anna Freud, argued back. She then sent those same nurses the literature she had been reading about child separation and anxiety, and wrote an article for the *American Journal of Nursing* about her experiences.[107] This article planted the seed for her PhD, which she completed at NYU in 1964. This work, a study of the effects of maternal attendance during hospitalization on the posthospital behavior of young children, led to major policy change in hospital practices around "rooming in" and helped her attain a grant from the NIMH to set up a child psychiatry masters at NYU.

In 1957 Ildaura Murillo-Rohde also returned to NYC and opened some of the city's first "walk-in" mental health clinics at Elmhurst General Hospital and Metropolitan Hospital. In 1964 she was one of five founding members (and the only nurse) who received money from the NIMH to establish the Family Therapy and Study Unit at Metropolitan Hospital, which went on to develop instruments for research and evaluation of brief family therapy and training.[108] In 1968 Murillo-Rohde opened her own private practice in marriage and family therapy as a certified member of the American Association of Marriage and Family Therapy, eventually becoming the first nurse to be president of the association.[109] Her work in family therapy was groundbreaking in its focus on addiction, same-sex marriage, single-parent families, and cultural and racial issues for mental health.[110] Murillo-Rohde is an exemplar of the first generation of graduate students who took their focus on interpersonal relations into family and community work, where they set about establishing truly autonomous practice models.

Interpersonal Relations in Society

While interpersonal relations had originally been developed in the context of one-to-one nurse patient relationships usually in a hospital setting, it proved particularly adaptable to the outpatient clinic or public health model in which the nurse was the primary practitioner. But the theory itself had always contained this social and family element. The purpose of psychodynamic nursing practice and psychotherapy was the prevention and resolution of individual and social problems of living. Psychiatric nurses had long claimed that their work had an inherently social purpose. For nurses, this belief fed into the development of outpatient and community clinics, and an interest in the role of mental health teams and the public health nurse.[111] Peplau argued that public health nurses had roles to play in the development of knowledge about the relationship between environments and mental health because "such knowledge will yield practices that are preventative of pathology, ones that constitute early intervention in relation to early signs of developing pathology."[112] This knowledge needed to be built with the active input of the nurse, who was in a unique position to provide data. It was only through the observation and collection of data and the generation of nurse-specific theory that nursing could develop its own program and advocate for its unique and special role, including in the area of health promotion.

In terms reminiscent of much earlier engagement with mental hygiene, Peplau also spelled out the usefulness of the public health nurse in "mental health promotion," arguing that she was already in a position of being well liked and respected by families, and well situated within communities to see problems as they developed. "The public health nurse is a known source of certain help; she is welcomed into homes and shops, she is given information about the stresses and strains that occur in the lives of people."[113] In this way the nurse could understand, observe, and collect data about family, social, and environmental issues that may have been linked to the development of mental illness, which could contribute to broader knowledge and the development of programs.[114] Social policy itself in the postwar era was driven by, and created, a thirst for new knowledge. As Robert Felix, director of the NIMH from 1949 to 1964 argued, the development of new knowledge and new practices depended in the first instance on the gathering of data, which was sadly lacking in the area of mental health.[115] Peplau argued that good nursing practice itself depended on the nurse's ability to observe and interpret data, and that this data "can be ordered into theories toward a science of nursing practices."[116]

Nurses' observations also needed to be part of a broader social project, involving the development of knowledge about human behavior. In 1956

Peplau argued that "one vehicle for collecting data needed for the study of social contexts in hospitals is developing in the form of nursing teams."[117] Nurses had a responsibility to use their position and work in hospitals to contribute to the national project, and Peplau made the broader purpose of nursing observations explicit: "In behavioral science there is considerable research going on in order to develop generalizations that will become laws of human behavior. . . . There is a gold mine of clinical data before the very noses of nurses and much of it is in the interpersonal area. Let's get to it, observe, understand it, and decide what to do with it so as to benefit mankind."[118]

In many ways, Peplau saw the ward as a microcosm of society, and believed that good nurses could and should use the observations they saw there to contribute to broader social knowledge about human behavior. "There is a trend well in progress toward placement of psychiatric units within general hospitals. This trend emphasizes the view that a more complete study of the patient as a whole can be made in a facility that has personnel and equipment for such comprehensive study."[119] This obsession with understanding human behavior in interpersonal relations stemmed from an urgent social need to understand aggression in particular, and to forestall conflict on both a personal and international level. It was essential, Peplau argued, that nurses incorporate this knowledge into their own practice not just for the good of the profession but for that of society more broadly.

Peplau's work was most obviously relevant to the small-scale inpatient institution. However, she was not unaware of the emerging shift toward community-based services. She argued that the nurse in a community mental health team would continue to play an important national role in research and gathering information because public health "agency reports provide an important source of data about trends in family life."[120] These reports, and the work of the nurse in families, were essential in helping to "reduce the incidence of mental illness (or at least hospitalization for mental illness), and the spread of this contagious socio-psychological disease."[121] The idea that mental illness was "contagious" is an interesting one, and was not confined to Peplau at this time. While it can be traced back to ideas inherent in the mental hygiene era, by the 1950s war experience had taught many mental health practitioners that soldiers' "breakdowns" were caused by environmental stress, and that they occurred more frequently in some units than others.[122] It was not so much contagious in a physiological sense, but inextricably linked to broader social circumstances and their stresses, from which no one was immune.[123]

Peplau's emphasis on the social context of mental illness reflected a general belief that it was only through the connection with broader social and cultural issues that the knowledge for advanced nursing practice could develop adequately. On one hand, Peplau argued that nurses needed to understand the social and cultural context of their patients, and to take that context seriously in the development of therapeutic treatment and care. On the other hand, her emphasis on the social aspects of mental health reflected her belief that nurses were an integral part of a broad social project aimed at establishing a functioning, democratic society in the postwar landscape.

Nursing for Social Change

The focus in nursing scholarship in the 1950s on the therapeutic function of the nurse marked a distinct shift in the conceptualization of nursing work, and not just in inpatient mental health settings. As Peplau recalled in her oral history, the idea of nurses as active therapeutic agents "changed the whole field of nursing. . . . In the 40s you couldn't have talked about nursing as the diagnosis and treatment of actual and potential human responses to actual and potential human health problems . . . the clinical specialist was really a silent revolution."[124] In this revolution, she saw the role of nurses as moving away from the paternalism of the "doing to" model to a "talking with" model—the goal being to achieve both the development and reflexivity of the nurse, and the self-development and self-empowerment of the individual.[125] Significantly, this development needed to happen at the patient's own pace and within his or her social system,[126] and it is in this sense that we see the power of interpersonal relations as Peplau envisaged it. Mental illness was a social problem because it occurred in, and was treated through, the relation of the individual to the family, and the family to society. Nurses needed to be cognizant of these broader dynamics in their own relations with patients and so their role was a social one as much as an individually therapeutic one.

It was in the application of interpersonal relations to social problems that psychiatric nurses undertook a power project as much as a knowledge one. While the initial attempts to reframe and transform psychiatric nursing knowledge had been about improving approaches to patient care and conditions within hospitals, the rapidly shifting terrain of psychiatric practice meant that nurses' impact on institutions was, in reality, minimal. The development of interpersonal relations as the framework for nursing practice had added legitimacy and authority to nurses as theorists, and had opened new avenues for practice. It had also opened debates within nursing itself about the nature of nursing care, and launched many psychiatric nurses into positions of power within nursing and mental health organizations. However, it was the capacity of psychiatric nursing to contribute to knowledge about human behavior and social problems that really promised to give the profession broader social legitimacy. As American society took a decidedly therapeutic turn in the 1960s, psychiatric nurses found they needed to engage with the complicated social contexts of their practice. Chapter 5 explores some of these social contexts and the responses of psychiatric nurses to the impact of social and political change on their theory and practice.

"The Number One Social Problem"

Mental Health and American Democracy

As psychiatric nursing grew toward the 1960s, its leadership increasingly engaged with the social and political circumstances of American life and its consequences for mental health. In a speech to the American Nurses Association (ANA) in 1958, Hildegard Peplau stated that "nurses outside of psychiatric hospitals have become aware of mental illness, not only as a major health problem, but as the number one social problem of our times."[1] In this speech Peplau made direct links between mental health and social stability, and argued that psychiatric nursing needed to be part of an active program aimed at ameliorating these social problems themselves through an understanding of human behavior. For nursing, this also meant facing the impact of those social problems on the profession itself. This chapter explores the impact of particular political and social movements on psychiatric nursing, beginning with an analysis of the focus on anxiety in the Atomic Age. During the Cold War in particular, psychiatric experts were quick to diagnose communism as a sickness, and to link the growth of neurosis and anxiety to postwar social change. Nurses made direct links between mental illness and authoritarian personalities, and argued that mental health was essential for American democracy. The fixation on anxiety, however, revealed the racial bias inherent to psychiatric practice, which saw social movements like civil rights and women's rights as causes of white anxiety.

Yet nursing was well aware of the needs of minorities as both patients and potential nurses. Earlier attempts at racial integration in the profession now extended to psychiatric work, and were not confined to northern institutions. The chapter also considers the relationship between southern and northern nurses in their attempt to navigate segregated educational and clinical spaces.

It then looks at specific projects in the South that sought to bring psychiatric services to southern patients and demonstrates the effect of the deeply held racist beliefs and segregated practices that undermined their efforts. Nurses were essential to both the upholding and dismantling of segregation in psychiatry, and their varied responses to the Civil Rights Act (1964) demonstrate the conflicting tensions that nurse leaders needed to negotiate well into the 1970s.

The Problem of White Anxiety

Throughout the 1950s, as Gerald N. Grob and others have argued, the psychoanalytic influence in American psychiatry had the perhaps unintended consequence of focusing mental health policy reform away from chronic illness such as schizophrenia (which was still not well understood and often dismissed as incurable) toward the "neurotic" illnesses, which could be "cured" through therapy.[2] These illnesses were seen not as organic but as interpersonal, stemming from fraught relationships and dysfunctional environments and causing ongoing "problems of living" in adult life.[3] Nurses actively pursued this line of thinking, and when social psychiatry intermingled with psychoanalysis, it too shaped the way that nursing knowledge itself would develop.

In the United States, the Group for the Advancement of Psychiatry (GAP), led by William Menninger, engaged in a protracted struggle to wrestle mental health away from a strictly biomedical model to a more psychotherapeutic one, and the influence of these ideas on public thinking and policy at this time was profound.[4] With their psychoanalytic focus on neurosis, the American Psychiatric Association (APA) and GAP were explicitly concerned with the problem of anxiety in the postwar era. Erich Fromm's book *Escape from Freedom*, which dealt explicitly with the "age of anxiety," was published in the United States in 1941.[5] In 1948 William Menninger published *Psychiatry in a Troubled World*.[6] The influential psychologist, philosopher, and professor at Columbia University Rollo May published *The Meaning of Anxiety* in 1950, and in 1952 the Social Science Research Council was funded by the Rockefeller Foundation to undertake studies in social psychiatry that might find solutions to the problem of anxiety-inducing social change, potentially forestalling future international conflict.[7] All this occurred in the context of continued global unease as communism flourished in Europe, bringing with it the threat of nuclear warfare, the reality of Cold War, and the hysteria of anticommunist sentiment exemplified by McCarthyism.[8] These were all problems that interested psychiatric and mental health practitioners at this time, as they sought to understand the motivations for individual behavior, to extrapolate patterns of group behavior, and to understand extremes in political and religious ideologies.[9] The importance of mental health for social stability became an overt political concern in times of crisis, and was actively linked in the public and psychiatric domain with democracy and freedom. As historian Arthur Schlesinger noted in 1949, "Anxiety is the official emotion of our time."[10]

In 1950 Rollo May made an explicit link between anxiety and totalitarianism, dictatorships, and communism when he argued that "in such periods, people grasp at political authoritarianism in the desperate need to be relieved of anxiety. Totalitarianism in this sense may have been viewed as serving a purpose on a cultural scale parallel to that in which a neurotic symptom protects an individual from situations of unbearable anxiety. With some very significant differences, communistic totalitarianism fulfils a similar function."[11] If communism then was a kind of collective neurosis, it might have been understandable as a response to postwar anxiety, but it was to be avoided at all costs in the United States. "Even if we should escape being confronted with actual death in a shooting or atomic war," May argued, "the tension in the cold war can be used constructively for building our own socioeconomic standards in the West."[12] While anxiety may well have been the precursor to communism in Europe, it could be relieved by the "pursuit of happiness" inherent in the American dream: democracy, prosperity, and consumption.

Peplau and other nurses read and overtly referenced May's work in *The Meaning of Anxiety* and used these concepts for an explanation of the link between mental health, citizenship, and democracy. Psychiatric institutions and the nurses who worked in them had an overt political and social responsibility. As Peplau argued, "Aiding patients to develop competencies essential for living with people in a democratic society is in part the day-to-day task of nursing services in the psychiatric setting."[13] For Peplau, therapeutic practices had a social function as much as an individual one. The aim of psychiatric treatment, as Peplau understood it, was to create a self-sufficient, responsible person capable of functioning within the social unit. The therapeutic nurse-patient relationship was necessary in order to model healthy interpersonal relationships, which were essential for continued growth and social stability. According to Peplau, "Any illness or difficulty can be utilized as an experience from which can be learned something that will strengthen the sick person and his family—in their ability to withstand stress and anxiety, in their level of skill in problem solving, and in their development of insights which are useful as foresight with regard to personal health in the future."[14]

Anxiety was a central concept within Peplau's use of psychotherapy in particular because it was understood as the trigger for neurotic and panic responses. In much of her writing, she stressed the significance of anxiety for all nursing settings and the need for nurses to understand its impact for therapeutic and preventative work. She believed that anxiety underpinned all mental health issues. "Most of all," she wrote, "mental health requires knowing when you are anxious, how anxious, for what reasons, and how the anxiety can be reduced."[15] It was this failure of knowing, of not recognizing triggers for anxiety, of not being able to "manage" that anxiety, which set apart those with problems of living as a form of illness. In clinical settings, she argued, this kind of anxiety led to severe panic in which rational, self-conscious thought and action became paralyzed or triggered aggression and self-harm.[16] In other settings, unmanaged anxiety could trigger problems of living that would stifle personal growth, affecting the individual, family, and community. "Anxiety underlies conflict; the concept of conflict also defines behaviors that can be observed as cues to the presence of anxiety," Peplau argued in 1963.[17]

Dorothy Mereness was also cognizant of the social context of anxiety. She argued that the high level of social and cultural anxiety at the time would have an effect on nurses themselves, and could limit their ability to make interpersonal connections and provide therapeutic care. Nurses, as people, were anxious about changes in society, and they could not help but be affected by the anxiety of the Atomic Age. They needed to be aware of this anxiety in themselves and manage the impact it might have on their work. "It is difficult and often impossible to help others with feelings of insecurity if your own are great," Mereness argued in 1958.[18] In particular, Mereness stressed the very real challenges the broader social context of the neurotic illnesses posed for social stability. "Today," she wrote, "the end of the world is not a rumor but a scientific possibility about which we are all aware and all justifiably concerned. . . . Our television and radio programs pour out information about the advances which are being made weekly in the abilities of the nations to destroy one another. . . . Underlying all of the other causes for anxiety in this anxiety riddled age is a realistic concern about the future."[19]

Mereness argued that those social forces were having a direct and destabilizing effect on people, and that nurses needed to take this seriously. In 1959 she argued that "the first consideration should be given [by nurses] to certain social forces within our culture. These forces originate outside the psychiatric situation but constantly and subtly influence every . . . individual's attitudes towards themselves."[20] These forces included the changing role of women, the opening up of education, the desire for upward social mobility, the rights of the individual in decision making, and "the generalized fear and unrest related to the atomic age which pervades the thoughts and feelings of all literate people today in relation to daily safety and the very existence of our way of life."[21] In these statements, Mereness acknowledges the role of social and cultural trauma on mental illness, and she repeatedly urged nurses to be aware of the "unconscious mental needs of people and how these needs are influenced by stress situations."[22]

Nurses needed to take care of this stress, Mereness continued, through family connections and making sure their own interpersonal relations were sound. But insecurity could also be exacerbated by broader social unrest, such as the breakdown of families and the changing role of women. The emerging women's rights movement may have caused some nurses to question what they were doing with their lives, and feminist theory threatened to shake the very ground on which nursing care was built. Mereness argued that nurses should see this as an opportunity to solidify their professional standing and take comfort in their work itself. She drew on Freud to argue that fear and anxiety could be sublimated into work and that nurses could find satisfaction in it not least because of the worthy social function their work served in the stabilization of society after World War II. She noted as a positive that "nursing as a profession usually contributes to helping the individual nurse feel that she has a significant role to play in mankind's ever constant march toward a more complete life."[23]

In this sense, nurses had a responsibility to work toward establishing stability in the broader culture despite the tumultuous environment in which they were attempting to forge their very new practice. Peplau herself clearly articulated the importance of mental health for democratic citizenship, making a direct link between mental health and national character. After the war, she explained, "you had all these veterans who broke down. And to think it was a part of the American character structure was abhorrent."[24] The war had revealed that emotional and mental vulnerability transcended traditional notions of masculinity, that even the best and bravest patriot was at risk. This did not mean, however, that wounded masculinity could be permitted to stand. Rather, it required that these men, these *Americans*, must be restored if they were to take their place as citizens. As William Menninger argued, the optimism that men could be cured coincided with a belief that they *must* be cured.[25]

Citizenship was, of course, essential for a functioning democracy, which would distinguish America from its communist enemies. Mental health was essential for democracy because it signified the use of reason, a mature independence, and a sense of responsibility to fellow citizens. Peplau took up this theme in her work when she argued that "mental health has to do with recognizing and respecting one's capacities and taking responsibility for their use and continuing refinement in the interest of the common good."[26] In this broad sense, Peplau argued that mental health was linked to underlying social factors that threatened national security and stability. "The widespread interest in mental health coincides with community concern for improved education, reduction of poverty, and amelioration of social problems of many kinds which provide the climate in which mental illness can occur."[27] Nursing knowledge needed to be grounded in this social context so that nurses understood the implications of their practice beyond the hospital door, and could make a meaningful contribution to the broad social project that was now conceptualized as *mental health*, rather than *mental hygiene*.

It is the case, however, that an observer could easily be forgiven for thinking that this was a singularly white project. Very little overt mention is made of racial issues and the developing civil rights movement in the nursing literature throughout the 1950s, despite the fact that psychiatrists and psychologists were essential to the arguments for integration in education and health care.[28] New initiatives aimed at addressing the mental health needs of African Americans in Harlem included the establishment of small clinics and an inpatient service at Harlem Hospital. Black psychiatrists and nurses were part of these efforts.[29] But racial segregation remained an issue in nurse education. Debates about who should serve in the U.S. Army Nurse Corps during World War II had forced nursing associations to deal with racial distinctions in practice,[30] but segregated hospitals and universities meant that undertaking psychiatric nursing as a specialty was still difficult for black nurses. This was true for nurses both in the North and in the South.

Psychiatric Nursing as a Segregated Profession

If psychiatric nursing appeared to be a white women's profession before the 1950s, this was partly because even northern hospitals and universities that provided psychiatric training were themselves largely segregated. The Intergroup Relations Committee of the ANA and the National Association for Colored Graduate Nurses (NACGN) were working to address segregation in the profession, but it was at times necessary for the NACGN in particular to remind institutions of state law forbidding racial discrimination. This was easier in some states than others, depending on local politics. In New York, for instance, the NACGN took on the New York State Psychiatric Institute (NYSPI) as early as 1942. Mabel Staupers, the executive secretary of the NACGN, corresponded with a young nurse by the name of Alma Jones.[31] Jones had come from St. Louis to work in New York City. She explained to Staupers that she had applied twice to the NYSPI to undertake their postgraduate course but had had no reply from them, so was working at Bellevue Hospital instead. Jones did eventually hear from the NYSPI and was called in for an interview, at which time she was given a blank application form to fill in. She was then informed that she had been refused admission on the grounds of race. Staupers wrote back to Jones, assuring her that "we shall work on the situation at the State Hospital." She hoped that Jones would be able to take the course one day, adding that "it takes a long time to change these reactionaries, but when enough people become interested they cannot stand the pressure."[32]

Staupers did not stop there. First, she wrote to William T. Andrews, who had been special legal counsel for the National Association for the Advancement of Colored People (NAACP) and was currently one of the few African American members of the New York State Assembly. She reminded him of a state commission hearing that had ruled that "the question of race was to be eliminated from city and state blanks." She told him about Jones's situation, and thought he "might wish to check on this."[33] In October of that year, Ruth Logan Roberts, who had been trained as a physical therapist at the Tuskegee Institute[34] and was chairman of the Citizens Committee of the NACGN at the time, wrote to Thomas E. Dewey, who would soon be elected governor of New York. In her letter she spelled out that African American nurses were being refused work and education at specialist institutions like the mental and tuberculosis hospitals, and argued that these "un-American practices . . . violate both our organic law and statutes." She reminded him that as governor he would have the power to end these practices, and wondered whether he would.[35] On October 26, 1942, state attorney general John Bennett, who was also running for governor, wrote to Roberts and noted that as attorney general he had already ruled that state training schools could not refuse admission to African American women. He also assured her that "as Governor I shall use the executive power to the fullest extent to enforce our laws against racial and religious discrimination. I shall be particularly careful to see that State Institutions set the example in this regard."[36] When Dewey became governor, he appointed Roberts to the New York State Board of Social Welfare, and was instrumental in reforming New York's approach to mental health. He also made segregation in state services technically illegal, so that the NYSPI was officially desegregated by 1950.

Columbia University's Teachers College (TC) was also an option for black women wanting to become psychiatric nurses, and it attracted nurses from both the North and the South. The second cohort (1949) of the new master's program overseen by Peplau at TC included women from ethnic minorities for the first time, including Ildaura Murillo-Rohde and Ruth Johnson, a black nurse who had been working at Bellevue Hospital. In 1950 a second black student joined the TC program, Naomi Perry, who had been working at the Veterans Administration (VA) Hospital in Tuskegee, Alabama. Murillo-Rohde was careful to document

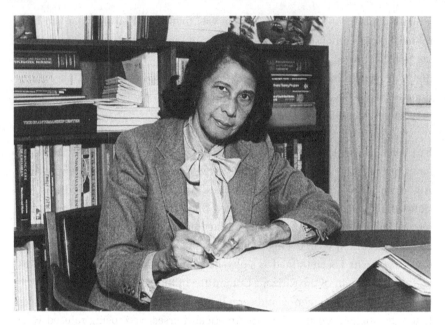

Ildaura Murillo-Rohde, 1970s. Photo courtesy of the Barbara Bates Center for the Study of the History of Nursing, MC 172.

the career trajectories of her Asian, Hispanic, and black colleagues who came through the TC, New York University (NYU), or Rutgers programs, and of those with whom she later worked or taught.[37]

Murillo-Rohde's cataloguing of names and careers demonstrated the complexity of the psychiatric nursing network across time and space. She also documented the intellectual work that nurses undertook in relation to the racism of psychiatry itself. Not only did minority nurses need to negotiate racially discriminatory barriers to their own education and professional advancement, they also needed to deal with racist beliefs about the nature of mental illness and its impact on their patients. Murillo-Rohde argued that "the tremendous social pressures, poverty and injustice" that minorities had suffered were directly linked to emotional and mental problems, and that "the mental health service delivery system has been insensitive and ineffective in meeting the needs of ethnic minority groups and misdiagnoses their problems."[38] She challenged the myth of emotional and mental difference in ethnic minorities and encouraged nurses to engage with literature that pushed back against these stereotypes. For Murillo-Rohde, more minority mental health nurses were needed not only to correct inequities and segregation in the profession, but also to represent for minority mental health needs. These needs often stemmed from the trauma of being a minority in America and the day-to-day reality of structural racism. This racism had underpinned historical beliefs about the inferiority of the nonwhite psyche, which led to abuse and denied them equal services. Murillo-Rohde spoke bluntly when she surveyed the literature, which proved "that ethnic minority patients are more often diagnosed as schizophrenics, are more often hospitalized and more treated with somatic therapies." In contrast, she argued, "whites are more apt to be treated in outpatient facilities, schizophrenia or psychotic diagnosis is less often used and are more often treated with psychotherapy. In many areas of the country, ethnic minority patients who become mentally ill were not only misdiagnosed, given excessive somatic therapies, denied psychotherapy as treatment and segregated in hospitals and clinics. But they were not treated at all in many occasions and subjected to custodial care as the only treatment."[39]

These circumstances were not ancient history; they were part of the everyday fabric of American life. This bias was "built into the mental health care system, and the profession of psychiatry . . . [, which] follow the path established by society at large. This is ingrained in the social and life fabric of our country if we want to admit it or not. It is sad but true."[40] For Murillo-Rohde, the situation would only change when more minority nurses became qualified to work in these systems and to bring culturally appropriate approaches to the treatment of minority patients. "More opportunities for graduate preparation in psychiatric nursing must be made available to ethnic minority nurses," she insisted. "They could be a great force and asset in the struggle to combat prejudice and to improve the care of ethnic minority psychiatric patients. They could be patient advocates to insure that the rights of all patients are respected and protected."[41]

At the same time as she called for more minority nurses to enter the profession, Murillo-Rohde was clearly aware of the obstacles and challenges that they faced. In her cataloguing of minority students, she was clear about how many had come from the South to study because they had not been allowed to join their state nursing associations or had been excluded from segregated nursing schools. Dr. Elizabeth Carnegie, dean of Florida A&M University's School of Nursing, had been frustrated about the need for her students to do their psychiatric nursing affiliation at the VA Hospital in Tuskegee, while Dean Lillian Harvey at the Tuskegee Institute School of Nursing also struggled to find affiliations for her students. Some affiliated with the VA but others went north to Crownsville in Maryland, or to Bellevue in New York. At Bellevue, they were joined by African American nurses from the historically black colleges and universities (HBCUs) Dillard University in Louisiana, Grady Hospital School of Nursing in Atlanta, and St. Phillips Hospital School in Virginia. As Murillo-Rohde documented, many of Tuskegee's student nurses chose to stay in the

North to pursue graduate study in these new psychiatric nursing graduate programs like the ones being established at TC and NYU. At the same time, she
was sure "that the racism and discrimination in the South that made it necessary for student nurses to go all the way to New York and other northern and
western states for psychiatric experience had to effect their desire to go into psychiatric nursing as graduates since they would not be permitted to work in
their home states in psychiatric hospitals. Some of the Dillard graduates returned
to Bellevue Psychiatric Hospital to work as staff nurses and later instructors in
psychiatric nursing."[42]

For nurses training at the Tuskegee Institute in Alabama, prospects for psychiatric work were marginally improved by the presence of mental health services at the institute and at the VA, which housed a mental hygiene clinic. First
funded in 1939 but put on hold due to the pressures of World War II, the Tuskegee Mental Hygiene Clinic became a community-facing mental health service
in 1948. The clinic was linked to both the institute and the Tuskegee Veterans
Administration in that it was overseen by Dr. Eugene Dibble (from the institute
and its hospital, the John A. Andrew Memorial Hospital) and Dr. Prince Barker
(a psychiatrist at the Tuskegee VA). It was staffed by Barker, a psychiatric social
worker, and some student nurses. The psychiatry program at the VA had a proud
history of paying special attention to the needs of African Americans in the
South. In the 1920s, the then clinical director Dr. George Moore (who had come
to Tuskegee from Meharry where he had been professor of nervous and mental
diseases) conducted research into the relationship between the misdiagnosis of
"Negro psychosis" and a hostile living environment, and argued that African
American psychology could not be understood separately from the social conditions in which people lived.[43] After World War II, the Tuskegee VA employed
some of the nation's most innovative black psychiatrists, men like Moore, George
Branche, and Charles Proudhomme, who went on to qualify as a psychoanalyst.[44] In 1962 Dr. Barker wrote about his experiences at the Tuskegee VA (from
where he retired in 1959). He noted that the staff was still predominately black,
but that the hospital had had two white nurses on the Medical Service, and
employed a white male attendant. He noted that desegregation of staff by the
VA meant that opportunities outside the South were being opened to African
American practitioners, but this would also make it "increasingly difficult to
staff Tuskegee exclusively with Negro physicians,"[45] who could find better paid
work in less stifling social conditions outside Alabama.

Psychiatric nursing was part of the Tuskegee Institute School of Nursing's
baccalaureate program, which had commenced in 1948 (the only bachelor's program in Alabama),[46] but aside from the VA, Dean Harvey was faced with the

very real difficulty of finding clinical placements for her students, and then places of employment when they had graduated. All other hospitals and colleges in that state were firmly segregated, and, as in most other states in the South, psychiatric services generally were underfunded and understaffed. Segregation exacerbated existing structural problems for both patients and the profession. For patients, it meant the continuation of separate and unequal facilities that led to abuse, neglect, and invisibility based on racist beliefs about the inferiority of the black psyche. For aspiring professionals, it meant limited education and training opportunities that restricted social mobility and the chance to provide services to their own communities. As the civil rights movement gained momentum, these combined problems led to national concerns about the "backwardness" of the South and the potential for social unrest. It was with these issues in mind that the Southern Regional Education Board (SREB) turned its attentions to mental health in the South.

The Southern Regional Education Board

After World War II, the economic and cultural conditions of the South were a concern for national stability. In 1948 sixteen governors across the South combined to form the SREB, designed to "uplift the South" through a collaborative focus on education and research. The main areas of focus for the SREB were the training of health, engineering, and teaching professionals, and it established separate program areas to identify needs and develop projects in each area. Two areas overlapped in relation to nursing: the Graduate Nurse Program and the Mental Health Training and Research Project.[47] The money available through National Institute of Mental Health (NIMH) grants had started to transform psychiatric practice in northern hospitals and universities and had already been used to establish advanced practice courses for nurses. Southern institutions were slow to avail themselves of these resources on an individual basis, but by late 1953 the SREB had obtained a grant from the NIMH to establish the Mental Health Training and Research Project, and had appointed Dr. Nicholas Hobbs from Peabody College in Nashville as the initial project director.[48] The objective of the overall project was broad, and the end goal was explicitly stated as improvement in patient care: "The payoff of the project will lie in improved care and quicker recovery of the mentally ill and in the prevention of mental illness (with the objective being) . . . to strengthen programs of mental health through increasing the number and quality of personnel and the scope and quality of research which contribute to the solution of mental health problems."[49] The project sat under a larger supervisory group called the Commission on Mental Health, which identified four professional areas to focus on: psychiatry, psychology, psychiatric social work, and psychiatric nursing. Both the commission and project drew on the expertise of people in each of these fields: "staff consultants" and "commission consultants," as well as state representatives.[50]

Even though the SREB was situated in Atlanta, the leadership of the mental health project came from Tennessee. Nashville was home to Frank Luton, one of the major innovators in psychiatry in the South and chair of Vanderbilt University's Department of Psychiatry, and also to Charles S. Johnson, renowned author, activist, and sociologist who, as president of Fisk University, was a tireless advocate for the desegregation of education in the South. The original commission consultants in 1954 also included Rufus Clement, president of Atlanta University, and in its second year it added Whitney Young, who had just been appointed dean of social work at Atlanta University.[51] Young in particular was an interesting addition. He had come to Atlanta from Nebraska, where he had been president of the Omaha branch of the National Urban League, and he went on to become executive director of the national body, as well as the president of the Georgia chapter of the NAACP. It would be naïve to assume this meant the SREB was looking to proactively further the cause of African Americans with mental illness, but it does reflect a federal legislative environment in which segregation could no longer be ignored. The other consultants to the commission and state representatives on the project were all white, and included Robert Felix, the director of the NIMH, Senator Lister Hill of Alabama (sponsor of the Hill Burton Act which had allowed segregation in Federally funded medical facilities) and Judge George Wallace, also from Alabama, who would later become governor and a notorious advocate of segregation in that state.[52]

Nurses were vaguely represented in the early stages in that Virginia Crenshaw from Vanderbilt was one of the original staff consultants, but it was not until mid-1954 that psychiatric nurses became part of the official project team. Some other familiar northern names appeared: Kathleen Black from the National League for Nursing Education (NLNE) was appointed as commission consultant, mostly because she was chair of the NLNE's section on psychiatric nursing; and Laura Fitzsimmons, the original nurse consultant to the APA and now chief of psychiatric nursing in the Georgia VA, was also appointed in 1954. The first task of this small group was to compile reports from each state on the status of education, training, and employment of psychiatric nurses, and to compile a list of issues and strategies. These issues and strategies would be discussed with an invited group of nurses at the first conference of the Mental Health Training and Research Project in Atlanta in July 1954.[53]

However, it had not been smooth sailing to get nursing participation or leadership within the broader mental health project. In May 1954 Esther Garrison,

head of the Nurse Training and Standards branch of the NIMH, wrote to Hildegard Peplau, who would be replacing Kathleen Black as the NLNE's psychiatric
nursing consultant. In her letter, she expressed pleasure that Peplau was coming to the July conference, and explained what had been happening behind the
scenes at the SREB:

> To begin with they have had no qualified psychiatric nursing consulta-
> tion and here they are trying to plan for education and research in the
> south with no notion (about psychiatric nursing) of 1) what it is, 2) on
> what levels it operates, 3) who is involved, 4) how to educate them
> (nurses in this instance although psychiatric social workers in some of
> the same dilemma) and 5) how much it will cost each year taking a long
> term point of view, allowing for development and expansion. They even
> asked for a definition of psychiatric nursing. None were in on the plan-
> ning and there was some half-baked notion that the 4 or 5 psychiatric
> nursing educators and a few psychiatrists might meet and make the plans.
> This is how I got in on it, screaming, with both feet, so here we are.[54]

In July 1954 the entire Mental Health Research and Training Project met at
the Biltmore Hotel in Atlanta. This conference saw all of the consultants, commission and state representatives, and representatives from each of the four tar-
geted professions meet together for the first time. The various professions broke
out separately to discuss issues specific to them before reporting back to the
larger group. Of the 150 people present, there were sixteen nurses, Esther Garrison from the NIMH, Kathleen Black from the NLNE, Hildegard Peplau, and
then nurses representing various schools of nursing across the South, including Emory in Atlanta, Louisiana State, Vanderbilt in Tennessee, and Duke in
North Carolina. Other attendees came from state mental health departments,
hospital education schools, or the VA and included Laura Fitzsimmons and
Mary Starke Harper, assistant chief of nursing education at the Tuskegee VA.
The group started its work by addressing issues that were pressing for most
nurses working in psychiatry in the early 1950s. Facilitated by Peplau, the group
asked her, and each other, questions that they struggled with in their day-to-
day practice, and they took advantage of Peplau's presence to explore theoretical and practical issues. Each question was presented to Peplau on a small note
card, and demonstrated a deep engagement with emerging nurse-specific theory in psychiatry, as well as a commitment to improving patient care. Questions
ranged from the practical, such as "How can the nurse stimulate better relationships between her and the physician so that all of the needs of the patient are
met, such as explaining reasons for new medications or treatments?," to the

structural, such as "Where is the dividing line between nursing practice and the practice of medicine?" "What part does hospital administration play in producing anxiety on the part of the staff?," to the deeply philosophical, such as "How can one attempt to relieve anxiety in a patient when the cause is a physical disability which cannot be resolved?"[55]

In asking these questions, southern nurses demonstrated they had the same practical and theoretical concerns as northern nurses, and the same commitment to improving patient care. Discussion of these questions and problems led to a series of recommendations that aimed to address the shortcomings in both the volume and nature of psychiatric nurse education, with the overt goal being the improvement of patient care. Participants made it clear that they needed support from their heads of school and state nursing associations to make psychiatry an essential part of nursing education, and to develop specific programs for advanced education. These programs needed to be aimed at the development of independent nursing research studies, and at a practice that was interdisciplinary, therapeutic, and rehabilitative: "To meet the need for well-prepared psychiatric nurses in the Southern region, nurses' training and research programs should be developed as rapidly as possible. Preparation in programs which are conceived creatively and which explore and develop new and useful knowledge and expert competence in psychiatric nursing will enable graduates of such programs to function collaboratively in an interdisciplinary approach to the solution of mental health needs of the south." In their call for programs that should be twelve to fifteen months long, southern nurses registered their interest in theory "of a most modern type" that would also enable them to develop research studies that would "extend the borders of current preventive, therapeutic and rehabilitative efforts in nursing and in its relation to interdisciplinary mental health action."[56]

The recommendations of the nursing group were ambitious, but not surprising. They reflected the arguments and debates that nurses had been having for almost twenty years, and drew on ideas for programs already underway in the North. Discussions made direct references to the definitions of psychiatric nursing that the NLNE had developed in its earlier work, and participants used the Claire Mintzer Fagin study (see chapter 4) to map out the deficiencies and requirements for nurse workforces in the South. They would not be easy to implement, however. The South was not merely lacking in workforce, funding, and infrastructure, but potentially also in willingness. After the conference, Crenshaw from Vanderbilt wrote to Peplau, expressing her hopes and fears. "I think we owe you a large debt of gratitude for all you did at the Conference in Atlanta," she wrote. "I don't know how best to express it but I hope future actions and time will tell. Personally, I think we would have come up with nothing much, had it not been for you and Esther."[57] And while the recommendations included overt references to the specific needs of the South, there was no overt discussion of racial issues. The silence is telling, and is highlighted by a small handwritten note in Peplau's papers. Tucked in with the conference materials, Peplau had kept a scrap of paper on which was written "The SREB staff have arranged for a special luncheon for a negro [sic] and white group at noon. You and Mary Scott and I are included—maybe others. They asked me to contact you. We are to meet in the ballroom entrance at 12:30."[58] There was no signature, and there is no further reference to this meeting in Peplau's files. It clearly indicates however, that issues relevant to African American nurses and their patients were on the agenda of southern nurses, and becoming obvious to their northern colleagues.

This July conference was just the beginning. The recommendations from each professional group formed part of the broader report of the Mental Health Research and Training Project that was delivered to the Governor's Conference of the SREB, which met in Florida in November 1954. At that conference, the governors were presented with the issues and strategies that each of the groups at the July conference had compiled, and agreed to proceed with the recommendations by appropriating $8,000 from each state budget to supplement the $73,000 the SREB had been granted from the NIMH. A formal council was formed with representatives from each of the four professions, and Peplau was appointed as the nursing representative, which saw her travel to Atlanta frequently over the next few years. Each professional stream then went about organizing its own activities, meeting separately and then all together again at a number of conferences, panels, and seminars between 1955 and 1958, including a large conference in 1957 in Oklahoma specifically for the psychiatric nursing group. This conference covered a wide range of issues, with delegates broken into smaller groups to workshop issues of workforce attraction, retention, and role definitions; new approaches to nursing education and research; and new approaches to patient care, with a particular focus on the idea of prevention through a public health approach and inpatient therapy. Attendees displayed a high level of psychiatric theoretical knowledge, and all of them were concerned with improving their approaches to patient care through the overt application of psychotherapeutic techniques. The conference report listed forty-six broad recommendations (with many of these including subrecommendations), including an interesting one relating to the "Promotion of Therapeutic Optimism." In this recommendation, the delegates identified one of the main barriers to attracting nurses into psychiatric work as the "hopeless connotation

which has accrued to it in the past." Rather, they argued, students, practitioners, and even the public should be helped to understand that "there is a hope-
ful future in the prognosis, care, and treatment of the mentally ill."[59]

The conference itself, and the activities of the SREB, gave Peplau hope for
the future of psychiatric nursing in the South. After the 1957 conference, she
wrote to the SREB saying, "I think you know that serving on the mental health
council has meant a great deal to me. I think this regional effort has a very great
and long range significance, and that it harbors the possibility that ideas imple-
mented as actions indigenous to the needs of the region will lead us to new patterns for solving psychiatric problems."[60] Importantly, Peplau pointed out that
the focus should now be on the improvement of patient care. She finished this
letter by noting that "nursing has stayed at the 'talking about psychiatric nursing' level for too long and the experience I have had in such workshops indicates the need to move to the 'let's take a look at what you as a nurse are doing
with patients' level."[61]

To facilitate this kind of close clinical work, more intensive educational
experiences were required. The SREB itself was not designed to establish
entire graduate programs for nursing, but it could facilitate faculty and admin-
istrator collaboration, and it did this largely through its broader program on
"Collegiate Education in Nursing." This was a smaller group that had been
holding meetings from early 1951, comprising several SREB office staff and
key deans of nursing in the South. The group included Ada Fort from Emory
University, Florence Hixson from the University of Alabama, Florence Gipe
from the University of Maryland, Elizabeth Kemble from the University of
North Carolina, Alma Gault from Meharry Medical College, and, significantly,
representatives from several HBCUs, such as Rita Miller from Dillard, Mary
Carnegie from Florida A&M, and Lillian Harvey from Tuskegee. At a meeting
in March 1955 in Baltimore, this group agreed that the schools of nursing at
the University of Maryland and the University of North Carolina at Chapel
Hill, as well as potentially the University of Texas, would apply for NIMH
funds for graduate clinical specialty programs in psychiatric nursing, with the
intention that all the rest would follow suit when in a position to do so. While
these large-scale programs were in development, the group explored other
ways to integrate new psychiatric concepts into their existing education and
training programs. One avenue developed for this goal was the "Clinical
Aspects of Graduate Programs" seminar series, the aim of which was to "test
out and refine nursing skills and techniques in the framework of the overall
therapeutic process necessary for the improvement of patient care."[62] Twelve
participants were selected from the southern states, and the plan was for them

to meet regularly in the intensive workshops. The first workshop was held in November 1958 in Atlanta, and was facilitated by Peplau and Elizabeth Bixler from the SREB. One of the faculty attendees was an associate professor of psychology who had just been appointed to the nursing faculty at the University of Alabama. His name was Arthur Dohlstrom, and it is through his appointment and experience in Alabama that we can gain insight into some of the challenges faced by psychiatric nurses across the South.

Nursing and Civil Rights in Alabama

The University of Alabama's school of nursing and its attempts to introduce psychiatric nursing programs reflect the complex political and cultural forces that hampered attempts to provide improved patient care in the segregated south. Decisions made by the governors of Alabama in an effort to avoid racial desegregation impacted the ability of health care professionals to provide adequate mental health care to all the people of Alabama. The state was home to two large state mental health institutions: Bryce Hospital in Tuscaloosa (which also included the Partlow School for Children) and Searcy Hospital in Mobile. After World War II, the patient populations in Bryce and Searcy Hospitals expanded to a combined total of over six thousand. Bryce Hospital was largely reserved for white patients, although black patients numbering around 350 were housed in segregated wards and a farm colony. Searcy was for black patients only. Both hospitals were horrendously understaffed: Bryce employed on average three physicians who passed as "psychiatrists" (although specialist psychiatric training was not available in Alabama until 1956) and one PhD-prepared research psychologist; an average of about twenty nurses, of which five were fully registered and the rest "practical nurses"; and about five hundred attendants. Searcy had a single "assistant superintendent" and used the same medical staff as Bryce, and from the later 1950s began to employ Cuban physicians who were refugees of the revolution. None of these physicians were psychiatrists or licensed to practice medicine in the United States. At one point in the 1950s, Searcy employed merely three registered nurses (all white) and more than eight hundred untrained black and white attendants.[63] The issue for these hospitals was largely the lack of a student nurse workforce. Bryce Hospital was on the same campus as the University of Alabama in Tuscaloosa, which did not receive a charter for a baccalaureate program until 1950. This program took its first class in makeshift buildings on the Tuscaloosa campus, but most of the clinical education took place in Birmingham at the University of Alabama's growing medical center there. Hospital-based diploma students had minimal exposure to psychiatric work through a limited affiliation with the VA hospitals

in Tuscaloosa and Birmingham, and other diploma programs scattered throughout the state offered no psychiatric affiliation.

Through her participation in the SREB group on graduate education in nursing, Florence Hixson, the dean of nursing at the University of Alabama, was
encouraged to apply for external funding. In 1957 she applied for and was
awarded two grants from the NIMH. The first grant was to facilitate the employment of faculty qualified to enhance the teaching of mental health concepts
within the new school of nursing, and the school appointed Dr. Arthur Dohlstrom to the position of professor of mental health. Dean Hixson noted in her
annual report that Dohlstrom had a BS and MS in education, and a PhD in clinical psychology from NYU. He had been working already in Alabama as the
clinical psychological consultant to the State Department of Mental Hygiene,
but his interest in nursing was genuine: at the seminar series he agreed with
Peplau that nurses had a significant therapeutic role to play, and he advocated
that the nurses in the SREB group meet together regularly to exchange new ideas
for research and practice.[64] Dean Hixson was glad to finally have some dedicated faculty in mental health, and saw his role as essential for helping "both
faculty and students in utilizing mental health concepts in the teaching and
learning processes and in the nursing care of patients."[65]

The second grant awarded to the University of Alabama School of Nursing
was for the establishment of a "Psychiatric Education" course for diploma students across the state. The course was to be run in conjunction with Bryce Hospital, and the chief nurse there, Ruth Oglesby, but administered by the School
of Nursing. The intent was for students across the state to attend twelve-week
intensive courses at Bryce, which would facilitate a coherent approach to the
teaching of psychiatric principles and the dissemination of the latest ideas. Hixson appointed Elizabeth Dutter from her own staff to be the project coordina-
tor.[66] The program expanded rapidly, replacing the School of Nursing's previous
affiliation with the VA, and students came from seven diploma schools of nursing across the state. The number of students enrolled in the program more than
doubled each semester, so that within three years of the first intake of seven students Dean Hixson could report that more than 170 students were enrolled for
1962.[67] The demand for this course grew so large that Hixson needed to offer
the course three times per year, instead of the original two, and she employed
two more faculty, both of whom worked part time in the program and then in
the School of Nursing itself. Hixson faced major challenges in her quest to find
and keep suitably qualified staff. Repeatedly in the 1950s and 1960s she wrote in
her annual report that while she was happy with how things were progressing
in the undergraduate space, she was also struggling to attract and keep suitably

qualified advanced practice faculty. She was usually able only to employ instructors who had recently graduated from their own program at the University of Alabama, and she often could not keep them in the state. The main reason she gave for this attrition was money; she was not able to offer faculty the same salary they would get in other states. In fact, in 1962 she lost both Dohlstrom and Dutter to universities outside the state because they were offered more than 30 percent more than what she could offer them in Alabama.[68]

In 1967 the School of Nursing joined with the Birmingham-based Medical Center and the College of General Studies to become the University of Alabama at Birmingham (UAB). UAB and the Medical Center were officially racially integrated, but Hixson could not secure NIMH funding for a master's in psychiatric nursing program until 1970 because she was unable to attract staff. When she did, she employed two women from outside the state: Cynthia Rector, who was a native Alabaman but had graduated from and taught in Peplau's program at Rutgers, and Arthur Ree Campbell, an African American graduate of the University of Maryland who was a certified psychotherapist. Interestingly, Campbell had earned her BSN at Tuskegee in the early 1960s, and she remembered her experience there fondly: "Dr Lillian Holland Harvey . . . was the dean there. I was fortunate to be there during her tenure. Or unfortunate enough, whichever the case may be, because it was a very rigorous program. And those of us that graduated considered ourselves to be among the elite and very blessed."[69] Even so, Campbell had needed to leave the state to advance her education.

Throughout the 1960s, Hixson repeatedly lamented the lack of state budgetary appropriations for mental health work. While the state appropriation was indeed low, the real problem came in the refusal of the state to apply for and accept federal funds. Large amounts of money were obviously available through the NIMH, and then through the Community Mental Health and Construction Act of 1963. This refusal to pursue federal funds was inherently linked to the states' insistence on racial segregation, which was not seriously challenged until late in the 1960s.

Title VI of the Civil Rights Act of 1964 made it illegal for any institution receiving federal funds to discriminate on the basis of race, and it also provided for Federal enforcement of that clause. This meant that the Department of Health, Education, and Welfare (HEW) was able to establish a Civil Rights Compliance unit, which requested that all health services provide written reports of their existing situation. Some states were less rigorous than others in their approach to this request. Alabama continued its fight against desegregation across the board by doing the bare minimum it could get away with. In relation to the psychiatric hospitals, James Tarwater, the director of the Alabama Mental Health

Board who was also superintendent of the state hospitals, requested that the various heads of facilities certify their compliance in writing to him. The response from nurses was varied. The head of nursing at the VA hospital certified that the Civil Rights Act made no difference to the functioning of the hospital, whose chief concern had only ever been for the patient.[70] The desegregation of that hospital was further attested to by the aforementioned Prince Barker, who was now its chief and certified that both white patients and white staff had been admitted and employed since 1959 with no adverse consequences.[71] Mrs. Elsie Smith, director of the aforementioned Tuskegee Mental Hygiene Clinic, certified that unit's compliance, stating that doing so signified no difference in the way the clinic had always worked.[72]

Others were less enthusiastic, however. For example, Mrs. Snow from the Visiting Nurses Association in Mobile reported that "there has never been any discrimination in our services as we serve all who need our help." She added, however, that "at this time we do not have any Negro nurses on our staff or Negro members on our board, we would not hesitate to hire one who met our qualifications nor elect one to our Board who met our standards or needs."[73] Of course these qualifications and standards were impossible for black women in particular when they stipulated lengths of high school education that were simply not available to African Americans in Alabama. This de facto segregation would have continued if it had not been for the newly formed Office of Equal Health Opportunity (OEHO) in HEW. In 1965, with the passing of the Medicare Act and the availability of funds as leverage, the office hired a series of general counsellors who inspected health facilities receiving or applying for federal funds and reported on their compliance with the Civil Rights Act. In January 1967 the OEHO sent its assistant counsel Marilyn Rose to inspect facilities in Alabama, which she found appalling. Her findings had triggered an "administrative hearing" in which it was found that there was no medical justification for segregation of staff or patients, and ordered that Alabama's federal funding be suspended. Outraged, Governor Wallace took HEW to court, at which point the NAACP Legal Defense and Educational Fund also bought a civil action on behalf of patients. In February 1969 Judge Frank Johnson ruled that segregation of both patients and staff within Alabama's mental health system was illegal, and he ordered the facilities integrated and that discrepancies in pay and conditions be addressed.[74]

Before the dust had settled on this case, however, some white nurses and lawyers took action. In 1970 Governor Wallace had ordered that more than ninety staff from Bryce Hospital, mostly nurses and psychiatric aides, be made redundant. Concerned for both their jobs and the implications for patient care, nurses approached some activist lawyers about the possibility of launching a civil action on behalf of their jobs.[75] Judge Johnson advised the lawyers that he could not hear a labor case, but he could hear a civil rights case. The lawyers therefore launched a civil action on behalf of patients, a case called *Wyatt v Stickney*. In the course of the hearings, nurses testified as to conditions and practices of which they were a part. The case rested on the failure to provide treatment for involuntarily committed patients, which lawyers argued was a breach of the Civil Rights Act. Johnson ruled for the plaintiffs in February 1972 and his decision set out in considerable detail the level of abuse and neglect at Bryce, Searcy, and Partlow Hospitals, listing pages of recommendations for improvements that became known as the "minimum standards."[76]

As a federal judge, Johnson's decision also came to apply to all state mental hospitals around the United States, who were now legally obliged to meet these same standards. Many states, of course, were not able to do so, and proceeded to close hospitals down instead. Coinciding as it did with the broader move for deinstitutionalization and community-based mental health, Johnson's decision had a profound impact on Alabama mental health services. The standards themselves were expensive and almost impossible.[77] In late 1972 the Alabama Mental Health Board convened a gathering of psychiatric experts from across the country to help them develop a transition plan to meet the standards. Included in this group were psychiatric nurses Hildegard Peplau and Grayce Sills. The group spent two days touring the facilities at Bryce and Searcy and going over plans for repatriating more than four thousand people into the community.[78] In the process, the commissioner for mental health admitted that he had thousands of people in the system who should never have been there, people who were homeless or poor and not actually ill, people with no care plans and no diagnosis, people who were worse off than when they had come into the hospitals, people who now had no life skills and nowhere to go.[79] The state had not received any federal assistance through the Community Mental Health Act (1963) and had spent ten years and millions of dollars defending segregation in mental hospitals instead of improving services.

There was little real impetus for change. Returning from Alabama, Peplau noted that the meetings "left much to be desired—the MDs couldn't keep an eye on the focus. None dared comment on the rift in top admin as to whether to get on with implementing the court order or to play the 'what if' game with the court."[80] In fact, it could be argued that Alabama continued to play the "what if" game with the court for decades. The final ruling that ended the *Wyatt v. Stickney* case and declared Alabama in compliance with the minimum standards was not handed down until 2003 by Judge Myron Thompson, Johnson's immediate successor in the middle district. Searcy Hospital was finally closed in 2012. "The New Bryce" (a much smaller 230-bed purpose-built facility) still operates in Tuscaloosa today.

Critical Intersections

The role of nurses in the history of psychiatry is plagued with the tension between ideas of care and control. This is nowhere more obvious than in the debates around patient rights and the intersection with race. Black nurses were largely excluded from a profession that was itself built on the idea that African Americans, and other ethnic minorities, were inherently psychologically inferior. Nurses' conflicting reactions to the needs of minority patients demonstrate the long lasting consequences of medical racism that saw the black body and soul as inferior and abnormal, yet deliberately denied that black mental illness might be linked to the traumatic reality of everyday life in the Jim Crow South. The hypocrisy of American psychiatry was starkly revealed at its intersection with civil rights. White people were deemed necessarily anxious about the social and political consequences of their lives, a problem necessitating the expenditure of large amounts of money and the search for prevention and cures. At the same time, black anger at injustice was framed as either pathological or criminal, leading to the confinement of people against their will while those with actual mental illness were either hospitalized in substandard conditions or left with no treatment options at all. Nursing leaders had mixed reactions to these political and social circumstances, at times both part of the problem and the solution. The profession itself was deeply impacted by racist practices, especially in the South where political insistence on racial segregation led to a devastating loss of funds and major delays in the development of advanced practice. In the context of a powerful civil rights movement, psychiatric hospitals became sites of contested ideas about the nature of nursing care and African American psychology, and challenged the racism of American psychiatry itself. Nurses' involvement in the process of desegregation reveals a complex network of relationships in which government, legal, medical, and community actors debated long-held justifications for segregation, and finally ended the practice in the nation's psychiatric hospitals. The formal end of segregation, however, was not enough to eradicate long-held racist beliefs about mental illness and minorities. The experience and work of nurses related to minority mental health in particular demonstrates the political expediency and ideology that has driven, and continues to drive, decisions about and approaches to treatment and care, and how some lives matter more than others.

"An Intolerance of Difference"

In 1963 psychiatric nurses started two journals by and for nurses: the *Journal of Psychiatric Nursing* and *Perspectives in Psychiatric Care*. In 1981 the former became the *Journal of Psychosocial Nursing and Mental Health Services* under the editorship of Shirley Smoyak. The research, theory, clinical practice, and politics of psychiatric nursing is now well supported by a vibrant and dynamic publishing milieu, with a plethora of journals, texts, conferences, and grant funding opportunities. Mental health nursing is included in most schools of nursing as a core undergraduate course, and nurses can now practice independently as a psychiatric mental health nurse practitioner, with advanced study available through the Master of Science in Nursing or the Doctor of Nursing Practice, as well as the PhD. Nurses now engage with the full range of scientific, biomedical, psychiatric, and psychological theories of human behavior and mental illness, and actively use theories and concepts such as therapeutic use of self, recovery-oriented care, the tidal model, trauma-informed practice, and adverse childhood experiences in their everyday work. In many ways, the idea that nurses can and should be therapeutic is now accepted without question.

At the same time, the spaces for autonomous practice have become limited by both politics and science itself. The increasingly biomedical focus of psychiatry opened up space for the development of the clinical psychologist, who is now the person most likely to offer traditional one-hour, talk therapy-based options. The idea of nurses as therapists was always premised on the closeness of the nurse to the patient, and the availability of patients in the institutional setting. Throughout the 1970s and 1980s, these settings were transformed at the intersection of exposés from journalists and conscientious objectors, the consumer/survivor movement, patients' rights court cases setting minimum standards, funding through the Community Mental Health Act and Medicare and Medicaid, and the fine tuning of psychotropic medication, as well as the shift of people with mental illness to small acute care wards or prisons.[1]

The chapters in this book have focused on what nurses themselves had to say about their role in the provision of mental health care. What nurses had to say did not always translate into practice, and to make a claim that the new knowledge that nurses developed directly improved patient care is beyond the scope of this book, perhaps of any book. There is plenty of nursing research that tries to make this claim but these studies usually only reveal how much remains to be done in an area of human health increasingly underfunded and overcriminalized.[2]

The history of ideas in mental health nursing demonstrates the persistence of the tension between care and control and the difficulty of its dislodging. We have seen in this history the ways in which seemingly harmless ideas about prevention and mental hygiene could easily slide into eugenics and the belief that some people with mental illness or disabilities should be sterilized. We have seen the way that these ideas led to many decades of confinement, neglect, and abuse, sometimes at the hands of nurses. And even when nursing theories were aimed at the improvement of those institutions, and of patient care, we have seen the unquestioned normalizing tendency that runs through psychiatric thinking: that there is a single human "normal" to which all should aspire, and that to be outside that normal is to be deviant, and other. This history demonstrates that nurses rarely overtly questioned the assumptions that underpinned their practice, even when they were well aware of the social context and the impact of political expediencies specific to time and place.

This history also demonstrates the importance of nursing developing its own knowledge, and highlights the processes by which nurses were able to take control of their own profession. In doing so, they articulated a vision for their practice that was centered on the improvement of patient care and emphasized the centrality of the nurse as a therapeutic agent. This was a practice that revolved around the deceptively simple idea of "talking with patients." This idea is especially salient now that psychiatric practices rely so heavily on medication rather than talking, and that most of American's mental health care has shifted to the prison system. Some have argued that if better care were provided at the community level then diversionary approaches could take effect, but this requires more than just funding; it requires compassion and empathy from front-line providers, and a tolerance of difference that current political circumstances and the unquestioning linkage of mental illness with violence and criminality make increasingly difficult.[3]

The almost-last word in this book belongs, as it probably did in life, with Hildegard Peplau. In December 1972, as the immediate past president of the American Nurses Association, she gave a very long talk at New York University's Distinguished Speaker Series.[4] In this paper she was intensely critical of the capacity of mental health nursing's knowledge and power to challenge the fundamental tension between care and control. She laid out the history of psychiatry as a continual move toward diagnostic control and a hopeless obsession with "cure," and made a scathing critique of the medical model and its one-dimensional approach to human health and illness. She argued that the obsession of psychiatrists and researchers with diagnostic categories caused more problems than they cured. "Diagnostic labels," she argued "particularly in the absence of known causes, tend in this society to be used as epithets to disparage people with whom one is in disagreement. . . . Unlike other medical diagnoses, such labels are thought to characterize the person—his outstanding behaviors. Behaviors not in accordance with social norms are called a disease. . . . Diagnostic labels for 'mental illness' not only stigmatize and disparage but also suggest a sick-role to be taken." She drew on the work of critical sociologists and antipsychiatrists like Erving Goffman, R. D. Laing, and Thomas Szasz to highlight the way that psychiatric knowledge was used as a form of surveillance and discipline "to the detriment of patients," and argued that improvements in hospitals had not gone far enough. "While there are some such institutions that have shown improvement of the physical plant in the last few years, the truth is that there are still many in which inhumane conditions prevail, unnoticed by legislators or the public."

In this paper, Peplau expanded on her earlier claim that mental illness was a social problem, but this time she argued that the problem was society itself. Rather than locating the source of social problems like alcoholism or juvenile delinquency within the individual as a patient, she now lay the blame with social discourses, arguing that the construction of human behavior as pathological occurred when it was politically expedient to do so. She concluded:

> But more than anything else, mental health is a relative matter—a judgment made by someone concerning the behavior of others. . . . Nor is this society yet too willing to live side-by-side with people too different from themselves—people who spend what money they have differently, or talk in a different idiom or language, eat different kinds of food, or have a

different skin color. These same social problems of contrast and intolerance of difference are acted out in communities and families and in this process some people get labelled mentally ill. These are the signalers of problems within our social system.

For all Peplau's efforts, these are not ideas a student nurse is likely to encounter today. Serious and persistent mental illness is real, but so too are the coercive practices and ideological discourses that create an intolerance of difference. A reflexive understanding of the history of ideas that informed psychiatric nursing in the critical stage of its development may provide context to continuing tensions, and reminders about the central role of the nurse in the improvement of patient care.

From Alabama to DC and Back Again

The Archives of Mary Starke Harper

Mary Starke Harper made an appearance in chapter 5 of this book, which notes that she attended the Southern Regional Education Board conference in Atlanta in 1954. I can only assume that she was one of the nurses who met privately with Hildegard Peplau at lunch that day; I have no proof. I went looking for proof (and did not find it) in Starke Harper's professional archives that are housed at the Barbara Bates Center for the Study of the History of Nursing at the University of Pennsylvania in Philadelphia.[1] The boxes were delivered to me with the FedEx tape from transportation still wrapped around them. Starke Harper passed away in 2006, and in February of 2016 it appeared I was the first person to work with these boxes. They proved to be an overwhelming testament to the intellectual life of a remarkable woman and a treasure trove of resources about the complications of race and mental health. These were the materials that Starke Harper had read and referenced in her decades of work, and they were voluminous. They were organized alphabetically by subject (but sometimes the subjects were repeated in later files), and they were not in any kind of chronological order. They appeared simply to be the unedited contents of her filing cabinets lifted directly into archive boxes. The covers of individual folders were marked in her loopy black-Sharpie handwriting but there was often no context for the material. I could not do them justice in a few short weeks, and my pages and pages of typed notes now present many editorial challenges because they are as overwhelming as the contents of the boxes and impossible to distill neatly. Yet the existence of these archives, and their contents, exemplifies many of the concerns of this book.

Starke Harper's intellectual work falls outside the strict timeline of this book. Most of her published work appears in the 1980s and 1990s, and is well known for its contribution to the field of gerontological and geriatric mental health. Less well documented are her thoughts about racism and psychiatry, yet this is the topic dominating the bulk of her archives. Most of this work she presented at conferences or workshops, or was used for policy documents and advisory papers well into the 1990s. It seems important to close out this book with some reflections from a woman who is, in her life story and in her work, the very example of the challenges and concerns faced by black nurses wanting to do psychiatric work in the United States.

Born on September 6, 1919, in Fort Mitchell, Alabama, Mary Starke grew up in Phenix City, Alabama, the oldest of eight children. After high school, she enrolled in nursing school at the Tuskegee Institute, where she earned a nursing diploma in 1941 and then worked as George Washington Carver's private nurse. After a period of clinical work at the Tuskegee Veterans Administration (VA) Hospital, Starke Harper earned a bachelor's degree in education (1950) and a master's degree in nursing education with a psychiatric nursing clinical specialty (1952), both from the University of Minnesota. She was the first black graduate of the school of nursing there and its first black instructor. She returned to the Tuskegee VA Hospital as nursing director and later became director of nursing education. She traveled north again to undertake a doctorate in clinical psychology and medical sociology at St. Louis University in 1963. From there, she went on to work in clinical practice in VA hospitals in Ohio and New York. In 1972, Starke Harper joined the U.S. Department of Health and Human Services in Washington, DC. At the National Institute of Mental Health (NIMH) she helped to found and eventually ran the Center for the Study of Minority Group Mental Health Programs, and then ran a division for research programs on mental health in long-term care facilities. She worked with four consecutive presidents, providing policy advice and consulting to Presidential Mental Health Commissions and the White House Conference on Aging.

Some have argued that it was Starke Harper's experience as a student nurse and her unknowing involvement with the Tuskegee Syphilis study that led to her concerns with ethics and disparities in health care.[2] But I think this is to draw too straight an arrow. If, as she states, she did not know that her student work at the Tuskegee Institute was unethical in this way,[3] then it is more likely that her everyday experience with and observation of the poverty and neglect of the rural black elderly was decisive. Combined with her own experience as a young black woman trying to pursue advanced study and a career, Starke Harper was all too aware of the continued reality of racism in the American health

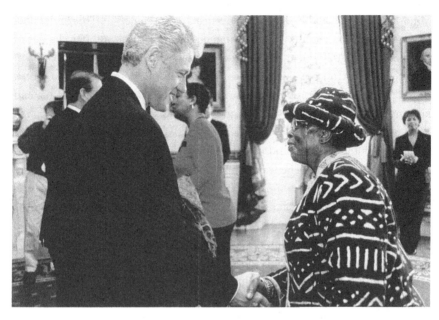

Mary Starke Harper with President Bill Clinton, White House Conference on Health Care Reform, 1993. Photo courtesy of the Barbara Bates Center for the Study of the History of Nursing, MC 150.

care system. Her archives reveal both her own experiences with this system and her deeply researched ideas about its impact on society's most vulnerable.

In her own career trajectory, Starke Harper epitomizes the experience of southern black women wanting to do psychiatric work. Unable to undertake graduate study in Alabama, she was forced to leave the state and become the first of her kind in northern states. Armed with a PhD, she was employed as the director of nursing research at the Montrose VA Hospital in New York. Here, she undertook a study of 147 patients comparing their diagnosis and progress by conflict (World War II, the Cold War, Korean War, and Vietnam War) and by ethnicity. She conducted extensive interviews with the patients and ran a statistical analysis in an attempt to understand the links between ethnicity, theater of war, and psychiatric recovery, and presented her work at the VA Studies in Psychiatry Conference in Texas in 1970.[4] When she applied for promotion, her letters of recommendation from senior psychiatrists were stellar, extolling her intellectual and clinical work. Yet she was denied promotion by an administration that cited a lack of clinical publication.[5]

In a folder labeled "NIMH Workshop for Minority Fellowship Program Interns," there are letters, memos, and forms not related to NIMH Fellowship workshops at all, but to her own struggle within the Center for the Study of

Minority Group Mental Health Programs to achieve promotion. This folder documents a yearlong conflict with her immediate supervisor and her charges of racism, ageism, and sexism.[6] The dispute was eventually resolved in her favor, and other files in this box document her extensive work in promoting the center, organizing grant application reviews, awarding and administering grants, and keeping statistics about the types of grants and personnel they supported. She identified gaps in the research program, and actively sought to connect nurses' projects with the center's funding.[7] Her colleague Shirley Smoyak told me in a phone conversation that she was responsible for awarding more than ten thousand fellowships for the training of health professionals to work in minority mental health. Smoyak told me that she would ring her at Rutgers (where Smoyak worked with Peplau) and say, "You must have some nurses there that want to work in minority mental health, send them to me so we can fund them."[8]

But it was her concern for the rights and treatment of minority patients within mental health systems that informs the bulk of the material in the archives. Numerous files in these boxes show Starke Harper was concerned about the ethical implications of psychiatric practices like restraint and medication. She was particularly concerned with the combined effect of overmedication and physical restraint on older people, and argued that nurses needed to work harder in this area to ensure the rights of patients and provide more compassionate and therapeutic care.[9] She stressed that health care providers needed to understand that the elderly with cognitive impairment or dementia were not simply "mentally ill," and that large doses of haloperidol were not the answer for disquiet or wandering.[10] The folder that contains this speech also contains a number of research papers that demonstrate the overmedication of the elderly as a form of restraint, as well as legal articles that deal with the rights of the patient to refuse medication. She used these articles to document the difference in approaches between white and black patients, noting that blacks were more likely to receive excessive pro re nata (PRN) medication and at much higher doses.[11]

Each box I opened revealed the breadth and depth of Starke Harper's reading and research, all of which she used to demonstrate the intersections between ethnicity, poverty, and crime. In a paper presented at a conference in Virginia in 1976, she drew on extensive research to demonstrate these disparities in action:

In 1971, the admission to all psychiatric inpatient and outpatient services were at the rate of 1239.6 per 100 000. Non-white admission accounted for 757.9 per 100,000, which is 60% of annual admissions. The admission rate for non-white schizophrenia is about three times that for white. It is estimated that over half of the resident population of public mental health hospital is non-white, whose length of stay in the hospital is longer and length of stay in the community is shorter than that for whites. . . . Non-whites constitute 70 to 80% of the prison population in the big city jails in the US. . . . In 1970, the census found 2.1 million persons were inmates of prison mental hospitals, juvenile facilities and similar institutions to a large extent, unfortunately the civil-legal needs and ethical issues are not addressed and assessed. Almost uniformly, the institutionalized population is poor and non-white.[12]

Her argument in this paper was that members of this marginalized and increasingly confined population became easy targets for unethical research and clinical practices that were not documented or regulated. These practices were underpinned by racist beliefs about the nature of the nonwhite psyche, which meant that "blacks are more likely to be seen by paraprofessionals than whites" and "more whites than blacks were selected for insight-oriented therapy." Minority groups received "qualitatively inferior" or less preferred forms of treatment, and "in terms of alcoholism, whites were channeled toward treatment, whereas blacks were disproportionately committed to prison."[13]

In 1978, drawing on material from a special panel on the Mental Health of Black Americans for the Presidential Mental Health Commission, she argued that racism itself was a causal factor of mental illness: "It is largely the environment created by institutional racism, rather than intrapsychic deficiencies in black Americans as a group, that is responsible for the over-representation of blacks among the mentally disabled. The racist attitude of many Americans causing and perpetuating tension, stress and hostility is patently a most compelling health hazard for black elderly."[14]

Echoing the words of Ildaura Murillo-Rohde, and plainly stating that which white nurses could or would not, Starke Harper located these racist beliefs and practices squarely in American history. In a 1983 workshop at the University of North Carolina, Chapel Hill, she argued that "each minority elderly has a special history—a collective experience that has placed its members in their present position in the American social system. That special history differs from one minority to another, but in all cases it entails subordination. The particular process was different: conquest, prolonged conflict and expropriation in the case of American Indians and Mexicans; slavery and its aftermath for the black, and a transplanted European culture of racism in the case of all groups. For the elderly black, the subordination has been coupled with racism, discrimination, negative stereotypes."[15] Racism, in all its institutional, historical, overt, and covert forms, was the biggest cause of disparities in minority mental health and not race. The only way to deal with this for Starke Harper was to develop a research agenda in nursing that was also a social program. This should be, she argued, a program "which takes into consideration the culture, folklores, life style and the psycho-social-cultural context in which minority groups live in a capitalistic, political and racist society. We need more in depth studies of the underpinnings, dynamics, and impact of generations of exposure to oppression and racism in mental health in order to program for minority groups."[16]

These short reflections, while representative of core themes, barely skim the surface of the material in Starke Harper's archives. Most of the quotes above are sourced from the first three boxes I looked at, and reflect repeated themes in her work. The fact that she continued to write and think about disparities and racism in mental health in the same vein into the twenty-first century was particularly striking to me, and as I continued to work through each box I felt my heart grow increasingly heavy. It was a long, grey February in Philadelphia, and I left the archive each day to negotiate the icy streets with my head down. In Box 9, there is a draft of a paper by Mildred S. Cannon and Ben Z. Locke marked "Not for Publication" and entitled "Being Black Is Detrimental to One's Mental Health: Myth or Reality?"[17] Mary had highlighted these sentences: "Until recently, research careers have been virtually closed to blacks. More emphasis must be given to attract trained and competent black mental health workers to assume research careers, raise their own questions, and develop their own priorities."[18] I typed out this quote and underneath it wrote the following note to myself: "What has changed? Nothing at all? Why not? This is really the question nursing needs to ask itself."

Acknowledgments

My acknowledgments start with a confession: I am not a nurse. I am a historian who has been blessed to find intellectual homes in Schools of Nursing in both Australia and America, but I do not know what it is like to be a mental health nurse. All errors of interpretation and oversight are mine and mine alone. But I have been cared for by mental health nurses, and inspired by them. This book owes its origins to a wonderful mental health nursing team in the School of Nursing at the University of Wollongong (UoW) in Australia, in particular Professor Lorna Moxham who first talked to me about Hildegard Peplau, and who exemplified all the very best of what she envisioned. Thank you, Lorna, and your team for your care and compassion for your students and colleagues and patients, and for the work you do with Recovery Camp and beyond. To everyone at UoW who believed in me, especially Patrick Crookes, Angela Brown, Joanne Joyce, and Maria McKay, I hope this makes you proud.

This book took international flight due to the support of the Barbara Bates Center for the Study of the History of Nursing at the University of Pennsylvania School of Nursing. It was Professor Julie Fairman who first suggested I come to Penn, and she has been a tireless advocate and mentor. Professor Patricia D'Antonio has forced me to do and think and be better, and has been so generous in her time and energy. Both Professors Fairman and D'Antonio have been strong supporters of a nonnurse working in nursing history, and I would not be here without them. The faculty and staff of the Bates Center have been incredibly supportive and helpful. Tiffany Collier, Elisa Stroh, and Jessica Clarke assisted me in negotiating complex archives and made visits to Philadelphia easy and painless. Professors Cynthia Connolly and Barb Mann Wall, both at Penn and at the University of Virginia (UVA), gave early feedback that shaped this project and continue to be a source of support. Jean Whelan made me feel so welcome at Penn when I felt like a fish out of water; her warmth and kindness will never be forgotten.

I have been the grateful recipient of a number of grants for this work and have many archivists and librarians to thank. Monica Blank at the Rockefeller Archive Center helped me negotiate the treasure trove of material related to psychiatry and nursing, and I am very grateful for the Grant in Aid that enabled lengthy visits at surely one of America's most beautiful archives. I was also fortunate to be supported by a grant from the Schlesinger Library at the Radcliffe

Institute for Advanced Study and spent many happy days in Cambridge buried in Peplau's extensive archives, to which I have not done justice. The American Association for the History of Nursing continues to support my work, financially and otherwise, and I am the grateful recipient of an H15 Award. The detailed work about Alabama would not have been possible without the support of the Reynolds Finley History of Medicine Fellowship at the University of Alabama at Birmingham, but I would not know anything at all if not for the help of Peggy Balch at the Reynolds Finley Library and Tim Pennycuff at the University of Alabama Birmingham Archives, who bought me realms of material and told me where to find everything else, including the best BBQ. The archivists and librarians at the Schomburg Center for Research in Black Culture in Harlem patiently helped me make sense of the National Association of Colored Graduate Nurses papers and the technology required to read them. Joan Lord at the Southern Regional Education Board in Atlanta opened a door to a whole world I did not know existed, and various archivists at the National Library of Medicine in Bethesda helped dig up material long buried. Thank you to Dianne Gallagher and the Howard Gotlieb Archival Research Center at Boston University for their assistance with the American Nurses Association Archives.

Being a historian of nursing is a wonderful and sometimes frustrating experience made easier by a group of people I now count among my friends and family. First and foremost of these is Winifred Connerton. It is not often you find someone you can talk politics, history, knitting, and shoes with, and knowing that I had such a friend, who welcomed me into her family, made the move to Atlanta and the finishing of this book imaginable. Thank you, Winifred, and also April Petillo, for our online writing group that kept me focused and questioning. And thank you to Professor Sandra Lewenson and Dean Annemarie McAllister for the collegiality as we edited a different book together, and for the Tuesday nights spent in boutiques on the Hudson Valley, including the personal chauffer service to and from Tarrytown. My wardrobe thanks you too! There are so many people to thank in the wider American Association for the History of Nursing community who have always been so welcoming to this outspoken outsider: Amanda Mahoney, Lydia Wytenbroek, Erin Spinney, Dominique Tobell, Melissa Sherrod, Gwyneth Milbrath, and Brigid Lusk at the University of Illinois at Chicago, Professor Arlene Keeling and Mary Gibson at UVA, and all the people who have listened and given advice at endless conference papers at UVA, the American Association for the History of Nursing, and the American Association for the History of Medicine.

I have learnt so much from the international history of psychiatry network. Thank you especially to the participants of the University of Sydney Winter

School in the History of Psychiatry for their generous feedback and collegiality. Thank you to Hans Pols and Mark Micale for inviting me and for the continued support and mentoring. I am particularly grateful to Thomas Foth and Geertjie Boschma, and to the group of historians of nursing in psychiatry who met at the Institute for the History of Medicine at the Bosch Foundation in Stuttgart in 2015. Thomas in particular helped me clarify my argument and continues to push me to think better.

At Emory University I have been blessed with a group of faculty and students who welcomed an historian into a School of Nursing even when they were not sure what she did. I will be forever grateful to Dean Linda McCauley and Senior Associate Dean for Academic Advancement Sandra Dunbar, who went to bat for me and continue to make a space for history and the humanities in a crowded nursing curriculum. My colleagues at Emory who have moved on, Maeve Howett and Angela Amar, dared me to dream big and remain a source of friendship and inspiration. I am grateful every day to the other Emory faculty who support what I try to do and see its value, and keep reassuring me when I lose faith, in particular Kate Yeager and Lisa Thompson. A particular shout out to Dorothy Jordan, who is both a stylistic and emotional inspiration. Your calm presence and welcoming home have been a source of true solace. It is the students who make Emory nursing what it is, and I learn so much from them. They inspire me to keep checking my privilege, and to focus on what is important. Thank you for the friendship, laughs, and learning to all the students who work so hard every day to make nursing a better profession: Dylan Avery, Alex Interiano, Sasha Cohen, Tara Noorani, Sarah Febres-Cordero, Gaea Daniel, Stefka Mentor, Isai Flores, Laura Franco, Pele Solell-Knepler, and Jordyn Seidman, among others. I am proud to know you.

I am doubly blessed to be able to teach in the Emory History Department and am incredibly grateful to the support and guidance of Professor Joe Crespino and the friendship and collegiality of Professor Susan Ashmore and Dr. Astrid Eckert. Past and present Mellon Fellows Elena Conis, Sari Altschuler, and Daniel LaChance have carved a path and continue to help me along the way. Professor Mark Risjord in the Philosophy Department is a mentor and colleague, as are Deboleena Roy and Elizabeth Wilson in Women's, Gender and Sexuality Studies. I look forward to what the future brings for the interdisciplinary humanities at Emory, and I thank the Mellon Foundation for their continued support of this important work.

Emory has also been a source of significant financial support through a University Research Council Award. I owe a special thank you to Allison Adams and the Center for Faculty Development and Excellence who make so many opportunities available to us, and who gave me the money to hire an insightful developmental editor, Katie Van Heest. Katie's kind but rigorous comments are what made this book readable.

At Rutgers, I am extremely grateful to Peter Mickulas and Rima Apple who encouraged this project and took a risk on me. Peter's patience, clear direction, and sense of humor helped me stay on track; I continue to spell "behaviour" with a "u" and prefer cricket to baseball. In that regard, my deepest gratitude for the expert copy editing of Paul Vincent. Thank you also to the two reviewers for their insightful comments, and to Professor Jonathan Sadowsky and Professor Susan Reverby for continued generosity and collegiality.

There is so much support that goes into the production of a single book. I might spend days at a time hunched over a computer but I am never truly alone. I miss my Aussie friends and the long walks on the beach, but they were there at the beginning and they are still there now. Love and hugs to Jane Downey, Fiona Donovan, Zena Smith-White, Alison Parker, Beth Garswood, and Pru Sheaves who listen to me vent and do not take me too seriously, and who remind me that really, knitting is the most important thing in the world. Jane, I miss you more than words can say but you have been with me every day. My Atlanta friends have kept me sane and grounded. Thank you especially to Magalie Remy and Veronica Jackson; I am so glad you let me sit at your table. Lou Robinson and Bill DeLoach have quite literally made this last year possible with meals out, meals in, rides to airports, complex shared custody arrangements, swimming, bringing me mangos. I owe you a debt I can never repay.

To my sister, Nardine Smith, who came to stay right when I had torn a ligament and had three months to meet my deadline, who helped me with the laundry, and who took Cookie for walks—I would not have got it finished without you. And Cookie, my little feral ratbag. We who love dogs know that dogs are the best people.

Lastly, but not least, to the family I chose: Tracey Ashton and Trent Shepherd. Trent, you are my rock. I owe you everything.

Notes

Abbreviations Used in Notes

ANA American Nurses Association

APA American Psychiatric Association

DAM Papers BBC Dorothy A. Mereness Papers, MC 55, Barbara Bates Center for the Study of the History of Nursing, School of Nursing, University of Pennsylvania, Philadelphia

GAP Group for the Advancement of Psychiatry

HEP Papers BBC Hildegard E. Peplau Papers, MC 59, Barbara Bates Centre for the Study of the History of Nursing, School of Nursing, University of Pennsylvania, Philadelphia

HEP Papers SLC Hildegard E. Peplau Papers, Schlesinger Library Collection, Radcliffe Institute for the Study of American Women, Harvard University, Cambridge, Massachusetts

IMR Papers BBC Ildaura Murillo-Rohde Papers, MC 172, Barbara Bates Center for the Study of the History of Nursing, School of Nursing, University of Pennsylvania, Philadelphia

MCR44 Docket No. MCR44, U.S. District Court, Montgomery, Alabama, Civil Case Files, 74-C-0813, Box 149, National Archives and Records Administration, Atlanta, Georgia

MSH Papers BBC Mary Starke Harper Papers, MC 150, Barbara Bates Center for the Study of the History of Nursing, School of Nursing, University of Pennsylvania, Philadelphia

NACGN National Association of Colored Graduate Nurses, Schomburg Center for Research in Black Culture, NY Public Library, Harlem.

NLM National Library of Medicine, Bethesda, Maryland.

NLNE National League for Nursing Education

RAC Rockefeller Archive Center, Sleepy Hollow, New York

RF Rockefeller Foundation

RG Record Group

SAMHSA Substance Abuse and Mental Health Services Administration

SREB Southern Regional Education Board

UAB Archives University of Alabama at Birmingham Archives, Birmingham, Alabama

VA Veterans Administration

Introduction

1. Edward Cowles, "Progress in the Care and Treatment of the Insane during the Half-Century," *American Journal of Psychiatry* (July 1894): 14.
2. Philippe Pinel used the term *l'aliénation mentale* to describe the condition of mental illness as a separation of self; see Albert Deutsch, *The Mentally Ill in America: A History of Their Care and Treatment from Colonial Times* (New York: Columbia University Press, 1962), 91.

3. Edward Cowles, "Advanced Professional Work in Hospitals for the Insane," *American Journal of Psychiatry* (July 1898): 21–29; McLean Asylum Training School for Nurses, Massachusetts General Hospital, advertising brochure, 1880, National Library of Medicine, Bethseda, Maryland, HMD Collection; W6 P3 v.7481 box 2188 no. 9

4. Significant patient narratives have been published over the last century and the experiences of patients and abuses in asylums are well recorded in films such as *The Snake Pit* (1948), *One Flew Over the Cuckoo's Nest* (1975), and more recently in TV shows such as *American Horror Story: Asylum* (2012–2013). Martin Halliwell meticulously documents the depiction of illness and asylums in film in his book *Therapeutic Revolutions: Medicine, Psychiatry and American Culture 1945–1970* (New Brunswick, NJ: Rutgers University Press, 2013).

5. Jonathan Sadowsky, *Electroconvulsive Therapy in America: The Anatomy of a Medical Controversy* (New York: Routledge, 2016).

6. Ellen Herman, *The Romance of American Psychology: Political Culture in the Age of Expert* (Berkeley: University of California Press, 1995).

7. Susan Reverby, *Ordered to Care: The Dilemma of American Nursing 1850–1945* (Cambridge: Cambridge University Press, 1987).

8. Substance Abuse and Mental Health Services Administration (SAMHSA), *Behavioral Health Barometer: Indicators as Measured through the 2015 National Survey on Drug Use and Health and National Survey of Substance Abuse Treatment Services, Volume 4* (Rockville, MD: SAMHSA, 2017), 11.

9. SAMHSA, *Report to Congress on the Nation's Substance Abuse and Mental Health Workforce Issues*, https://store.samhsa.gov/shin/content//PEP13-RTC-BHWORK/PEP13-RTC-BHWORK.pdf.

10. Bureau of Labor Statistics, "Occupational Employment Statistics: 29-1066 Psychiatrists," https://www.bls.gov/oes/current/oes291066.htm.

11. Kathleen R. Delaney, "Psychiatric Mental Health Nursing Workforce Agenda: Optimizing Capabilities and Capacity to Address Workforce Demands," *Journal of the American Psychiatric Nurses Association* 22, no. 2 (2016): 122–131.

12. Delaney.

13. William C Torrey, Ida Griesemer, and Elizabeth A. Carpenter-Song, "Beyond 'Med Management,'" *Psychiatric Services* 68, no. 6 (June 1, 2017): 618–620.

14. Kathleen R. Delaney et al., "The Effective Use of Psychiatric Mental Health Nurses in Integrated Care: Policy Implications for Increasing Quality and Access to Care," *Journal of Behavioral Health Services and Research* 45, no. 2 (April 2018): 300–309.

15. World Health Organization, *Mental Health Action Plan, 2013–2020* (Geneva: World Health Organization, 2013), 9.

16. Gerald N. Grob, *From Asylum to Community: Mental Health Policy in Modern America* (Princeton, NJ: Princeton University Press, 1991), 53.

17. Robert H. Felix, "Mental Disorders as a Public Health Problem," *American Journal of Psychiatry* (December 1949): 401–406.

18. The history of psychiatry literature is large and growing rapidly. The main sources essential for an understanding of the changes to psychiatric workforces are Gerald N. Grob, *The Mad Among Us: A History of the Care of America's Mentally Ill* (London: Free Press, 1994); Grob, *From Asylum to Community*; Gerald N. Grob, *Mental Illness and American Society* (Princeton, NJ: Princeton University Press, 1983); Gerald N. Grob, "Rediscovering Asylums: The Unhistorical History of the Mental Hospital," in

The Therapeutic Revolution: Essays in the Social History of American Medicine, ed.
Morris J. Vogel and Charles E Rosenberg (Philadelphia: University of Pennsylvania
Press, 1979), 135–157. For the history of psychiatric ideas and treatment approaches,
see Nathan G. Hale, *The Rise and Crisis of Psychoanalysis in the United States: Freud
and the Americans, 1917–1985* (Oxford: Oxford University Press, 1995); Eva Mos-
kowitz, *In Therapy We Trust: America's Obsession with Self-Fulfillment* (Baltimore:
Johns Hopkins University Press, 2001); Joel Braslow, *Mental Ills and Bodily Cures:
Psychiatric Treatment in the First Half of the Twentieth Century* (Berkeley: University of California Press, 1997); Eric Caplan, *Mind Games: American Culture and the
Birth of Psychotherapy* (Berkeley: University of California Press, 1998); Halliwell,
Therapeutic Revolutions; John Burnham, ed., *After Freud Left: A Century of Psycho-
analysis in America* (Chicago: University of Chicago Press, 2012); Mical Raz, *The
Lobotomy Letters: The Making of American Psychosurgery* (Rochester, NY: University of Rochester Press, 2013).
19. Arthur Schlesinger, *The Vital Center: The Politics of Freedom* (Boston: Houghton
Mifflin, 1949); Herman, *Romance of American Psychology*; Andrea Friedman, *Citizenship in Cold War America: The National Security State and the Possibilities of Dissent*
(Amherst: University of Massachusetts Press, 2014); Michael Staub, *Madness Is Civilization: When the Diagnosis Was Social, 1948–1980* (Chicago: University of Chicago
Press, 2011).
20. Grob, *From Asylum to Community*, 80.
21. Staub, *Madness Is Civilization*.
22. Staub; Herman, *Romance of American Psychology*; Halliwell, *Therapeutic Revolutions*.
23. Hildegard Peplau, "Current Concepts of Psychiatric Nursing," speech given to the
American Nurses Association (ANA) Convention, Atlantic City, New Jersey, June 11,
1958, box 2, folder 30, Hildegard E. Peplau Papers, MC 59, Barbara Bates Centre for
the Study of the History of Nursing, School of Nursing, University of Pennsylvania
(hereafter cited as HEP Papers BBC).
24. Felix, "Mental Disorders as a Public Health Problem."
25. Herman, *Romance of American Psychology*; Halliwell, *Therapeutic Revolutions*;
Staub, *Madness Is Civilization*.
26. Adolf Meyer, "The Birth and Development of the Mental Hygiene Movement," *Mental
Hygiene* 19 (1935): 29–37; Hale, *Rise and Crisis of Psychoanalysis in the United
States*.
27. Halliwell, *Therapeutic Revolutions*; Hale, *Rise and Crisis of Psychoanalysis in the
United States*; Nathan G. Hale, *Freud and the Americans: The Beginnings of Psychoanalysis in the United States 1876–1917* (Oxford: Oxford University Press, 1971);
Burnham, *After Freud Left*.
28. While the distinction between psychiatry and psychology in terms of professional
practice is clear to us in the twenty-first century, this was not the case in the 1950s.
Psychiatry saw itself as a medical science rather than a social science, while psychology was situated within the behavioral/social sciences. The scramble for expertise in the period around World War II and immediately after meant that both mental
health professionals and social scientists experimented along a number of theoretical and disciplinary lines and were not concerned that a "social" element overstepped
professional boundaries. The social theory component and overlap between European critical theory and psychoanalysis (and the influence of those thinkers in the
United States) meant that psychiatry was happy to call itself a social science, or to
be used for social purposes as much as it was for medical ones. It was also the case

that there was no clear medicine of psychiatry at the time, and American psychiatry used its psychoanalytic underpinnings to make claims of expertise in many mental, behavioral, and social science areas. See Herman, *Romance of American Psychology*; Grob, *From Asylum to Community*.

29. Herman, *Romance of American Psychology*; Dennis Doyle, *Psychiatry and Racial Liberalism in Harlem 1936–1968* (Rochester, NY: University of Rochester Press, 2016); Halliwell, *Therapeutic Revolutions*, 24.

30. Herman, *Romance of American Psychology*.

31. Deborah Weinstein, *The Pathological Family: Postwar America and the Rise of Family Therapy* (Ithaca, NY: Cornell University Press, 2013); Anna Creadick, *Perfectly Average: The Pursuit of Normality in Postwar America* (Amherst: University of Massachusetts Press 2010).

32. Herman, *Romance of American Psychology*.

33. Tom Engelhardt, *The End of Victory Culture: Cold War America and the Disillusioning of a Generation* (Amherst: University of Massachusetts Press, 2007); Friedman, *Citizenship in Cold War America*.

34. Halliwell, *Therapeutic Revolutions*, 68.

35. Halliwell, 79.

36. Reverby, *Ordered to Care*; Patricia D'Antonio, *American Nursing: A History of Knowledge, Authority, and the Meaning of Work* (Baltimore: Johns Hopkins University Press, 2010); Siobhan Nelson and Suzanne Gordon, eds., *The Complexities of Care: Nursing Reconsidered* (Ithaca, NY: Cornell University Press, 2006).

37. Deutsch, *Mentally Ill in America*.

38. Grob, *From Asylum to Community*.

39. Grob, 97.

40. Jonathan Metzl, *The Protest Psychosis: How Schizophrenia Became a Black Disease* (Boston: Beacon Press, 2010), 81–82.

41. Barbara J. Callaway, *Hildegard Peplau: Psychiatric Nurse of the Century* (New York: Springer, 2002).

42. Hildegard Peplau, "Oral History, Psychiatric Nursing Career," ed. Patricia D'Antonio, 1985, box 1, folder 2, HEP Papers BBC.

43. Grob, *From Asylum to Community*, 121.

44. John Burnham, "The Struggle between Physicians and Paramedical Personnel in American Psychiatry, 1917–1941," *Journal of the History of Medicine and Allied Sciences* 29, no. 1 (1974): 93–106.

45. Andrew Scull, "The Mental Health Sector and the Social Sciences in Post-World War II USA: Part I: Total War and Its Aftermath," *History of Psychiatry* 22, no. 1 (2010): 3–19; Andrew Scull, "The Mental Health Sector and the Social Sciences in Post-World War II USA Part 2: The Impact of Federal Research Funding the Drugs Revolution," *History of Psychiatry* 22, no. 3 (2011): 268–284; Catherine Fussinger, "'Therapeutic Community', Psychiatry's Reformers and Anti-Psychiatrists: Reconsidering Changes in the Field of Psychiatry after World War II," *History of Psychiatry* 22, no. 2 (2011): 146–163; Raz, *Lobotomy Letters*; Grob, *Mad Among Us*; Grob, *From Asylum to Community*; Braslow, *Mental Ills and Bodily Cures*; Moskowitz, *In Therapy We Trust*.

46. Laura C. Hein and Kathleen M. Scharer, "A Modern History of Psychiatric-Mental Health Nursing," *Archives of Psychiatric Nursing* 29 (2015): 49–55; Christine Silverstein, "From the Front Lines to the Home Front: A History of the Development of Psychiatric Nursing in the US during the World War II Era," *Issues in Mental Health Nursing* 29 (2008): 719–737; Tom Olson, "Fundamental and Special: The Dilemma

of Psychiatric-Mental Health Nursing," *Archives of Psychiatric Nursing* 10, no. 1 (1996): 3–10; Patricia D'Antonio, "Relationships, Reality and Reciprocity with Therapeutic Environments: An Historical Case Study," *Archives of Psychiatric Nursing* 18, no. 1 (2004): 66–72; Patricia D'Antonio et al., "The Future in the Past: Hildegard Peplau and Interpersonal Relations in Nursing," *Nursing Inquiry* 21, no. 4 (2014): 311–317.

47. Callaway, *Hildegard Peplau*; Olson, "Fundamental and Special."

48. D'Antonio et al., "Future in the Past," 312.

49. D'Antonio.

50. D'Antonio, 314.

51. Karen Buhler-Wilkerson, *False Dawn: The Rise and Decline of Public Health Nursing, 1900–1930* (New York: Garland, 1989).

52. Elizabeth Lunbeck, *The Psychiatric Persuasion: Knowledge, Gender and Power in Modern America* (Princeton, NJ: Princeton University Press, 1994), 167–175.

53. Ryan Johnson and Amna Khalid, *Public Health in the British Empire: Intermediaries, Subordinates, and the Practice of Public Health, 1850–1960* (London: Routledge, 2012), 3.

54. Winifred Connerton, "American Nurses in Colonial Settings: Imperial Power at the Bedside," in *Routledge Handbook on the Global History of Nursing*, ed. Patricia D'Antonio, Julie Fairman, and Jean Whelan (New York: Routledge, 2013), 11–21; Patricia D'Antonio, *American Nursing: A History of Knowledge, Authority, and the Meaning of Work* (Baltimore: Johns Hopkins University Press, 2010); Julia Irwin, *Making the World Safe: The American Red Cross and a Nation's Humanitarian Awakening* (New York: Oxford University Press, 2013); Charissa Threat, *Nursing Civil Rights: Gender and Race in the Army Nurse Corps* (Chicago: University of Illinois Press, 2015); Karen Flynn, *Moving beyond Borders: A History of Black Canadian and Caribbean Women in the Diaspora* (Toronto: University of Toronto Press, 2011).

55. Geertje Boschma, *The Rise of Mental Health Nursing: A History of Psychiatric Care in Dutch Asylums 1890–1920* (Amsterdam: Amsterdam University Press, 2003); Geertje Boschma, "Community Mental Health Nursing in Alberta, Canada: An Oral History," *Nursing History Review* 20 (2012): 103–135; Geertje Boschma, "Community Mental Health Post 1950: Reconsidering Nurses' and Consumers' Identity," in *Routledge Handbook on the Global History of Nursing*, ed. Patricia D'Antonio, Julie Fairman, and Jean Whelan (New York: Routledge, 2013), 237–258; Pamela Dale and Anne Borsay, *Mental Health Nursing: The Working Lives of Paid Carers in the Nineteenth and Twentieth Centuries* (Manchester: Manchester University Press, 2015).

56. Sylvelyn Hähner-Rombach and Karen Nolte, *Patients and Social Practice of Psychiatric Nursing in the 19th and 20th Centuries* (Stuttgart: Steiner Verlag, 2017); Tommy Dickinson, *"Curing Queers": Mental Nursing and Their Patients 1935–1974* (Manchester: Manchester University Press, 2015); Susan Benedict and Linda Shields, *Nurses and Midwives in Nazi Germany: The "Euthanasia Programs"* (London: Routledge, 2014).

57. Michel Foucault, *Madness and Civilization: A History of Insanity in the Age of Reason*, trans. Richard Howard (London: Routledge Classics, 2001); Michel Foucault, *Psychiatric Power: Lectures at the Collège de France 1973–1974*, trans. Graham Burchell (New York: Palgrave Macmillan, 2008).

58. Metzl, *Protest Psychosis*; Daryl Michael Scott, *Contempt and Pity: Social Policy and the Image of the Damaged Black Psyche 1880–1996* (Chapel Hill: University of North Carolina Press, 1997); Gabriel N. Mendes, *Under the Strain of Color: Harlem's*

Lafargue Clinic and the Promise of an Antiracist Psychiatry (Ithaca, NY: Cornell University Press, 2015).

59. Dave Holmes and Denise Gastaldo, "Nursing as a Means of Governmentality," *Journal of Advanced Nursing* 38, no. 6 (2002): 557–565; Amelie Perron, Trudy Rudge, and Dave Holmes, "Citizen Minds, Citizen Bodies: The Citizenship Experience and the Government of Mentally Ill Persons," *Nursing Philosophy* 11 (2010): 100–111.

60. Thomas Foth, "Biopolitical Spaces, Vanished Death and the Power of Vulnerability in Nursing," *Aporia* 1, no. 4 (2009): 16–26; Dave Holmes, Trudy Rudge, and Amelie Perron, eds., *(Re)Thinking Violence in Health Care Settings: A Critical Approach* (Surrey, U.K.: Ashgate, 2012); Perron et al., "Citizen Minds, Citizen Bodies"; Holmes and Gastaldo, "Nursing as a Means of Governmentality"; Amelie Perron, Carol Fluet, and Dave Holmes, "Agents of Care and Agents of the State: Bio-Power and Nursing Practice," *Journal of Advanced Nursing* 50, no. 5 (2004): 536–544.

61. This is an idea that emerged in conversation with Patricia D'Antonio, and I am grateful for her help with articulating my concerns about the segregated nature of nursing practice.

1. "The Backbone of Every Mental Hospital"

1. Elizabeth Lunbeck, *The Psychiatric Persuasion: Knowledge, Gender and Power in Modern America* (Princeton, NJ: Princeton University Press, 1994), 167.

2. The abbreviation APA is used in this chapter to denote the association that had changed its name from the Association of Medical Superintendents of American Institutions for the Insane to the American Medico-Psychological Association in 1893, before changing it again in 1921 to the American Psychiatric Association.

3. Gerald N. Grob, *The Mad Among Us: A History of the Care of America's Mentally Ill* (London: Free Press, 1994).

4. Nancy Tomes, *The Art of Asylum-Keeping: Thomas Story Kirkbride and the Origins of American Psychiatry* (Philadelphia: University of Pennsylvania Press, 1994); Patricia D'Antonio, *Founding Friends: Families, Staff and Patients at the Friends Asylum in Early Nineteenth Century Philadelphia* (Bethlehem, PA: Lehigh Press, 2006); Geertje Boschma, *The Rise of Mental Health Nursing: A History of Psychiatric Care in Dutch Asylums, 1890–1920* (Amsterdam: Amsterdam University Press, 2003).

5. Moral treatment was explained by Pinel in his work *Traité médico-philosophique sur l'aliénation mentale* published in 1801. It consisted of the removal of restraints, and the removal of the patient to a quiet (preferably rural) setting, the use of a light diet and calm surroundings, gentle exercise and entertainments like reading and music, and limited freedom. Importantly it rested on the idea of treating patients with dignity, and having trained attendant staff who were capable of the same. Punishments and physical abuse were to be avoided, with the end goal being that the patient would come to "minister to himself," and learn self-discipline and self-control. See Albert Deutsch, *The Mentally Ill in America: A History of Their Care and Treatment from Colonial Times* (New York: Columbia University Press, 1962), for the development of U.S. approaches to moral treatment.

6. D'Antonio, *Founding Friends*; Patricia D'Antonio, "Relationships, Reality and Reciprocity with Therapeutic Environments: An Historical Case Study," *Archives of Psychiatric Nursing* 18, no. 1 (2004): 66–72.

7. Edward Cowles, "Progress in the Care and Treatment of the Insane during the Half-Century," *American Journal of Psychiatry* (July 1894): 21.

8. Grob, *Mad Among Us*, 92.

9. Cowles, "Progress in the Care and Treatment of the Insane during the Half-Century"; Tomes, *Art of Asylum-Keeping.*

10. Linda Richards, *America's First Trained Nurse: My Life as a Nurse in America Great Britain and Japan, 1872–1911* (Diggory Press, 2006). Richards was the first student to graduate from America's first Nightingale style nursing school, established at the New England Hospital for Women and Children in Boston, in 1870. Richards's interest in "mental nursing" stems from her early experiences at Bellevue Hospital in New York and she remained an advocate of the idea that mental and physical nursing should not be separated. Her ideas will be explored in greater depth in chapter 2.

11. Cowles, "Progress in the Care and Treatment of the Insane during the Half-Century," 22.

12. Cowles.

13. Edward Cowles, "Advanced Professional Work in Hospitals for the Insane," *American Journal of Psychiatry* (July 1898): 21–29.

14. McLean Asylum Training School for Nurses, Massachusetts General Hospital, advertising brochure, 1880, National Library of Medicine, Bethseda, Maryland. HMD Collection; W6 P3 v.7481 box 2188 no. 9 gt.

15. A. B. Richardson, "Nurses in Hospitals for the Insane," *American Journal of Psychiatry* (October 1902): 225–232.

16. Given that Richardson's hospital ran its own training school it is unclear whether he means "registered" nurses from external schools, or graduates of his own hospital school.

17. Richardson, "Nurses in Hospitals for the Insane," 230.

18. Richardson, 225–232.

19. Richardson, 227.

20. Lunbeck, *Psychiatric Persuasion*, 172.

21. Charles Bancroft, "Women Nurses on Wards for Men in Hospitals for the Insane," *American Journal of Psychiatry* (October 1906): 177–189.

22. Bancroft.

23. Bancroft.

24. Richardson, "Nurses in Hospitals for the Insane," 231.

25. Richardson, 229.

26. Lunbeck, *Psychiatric Persuasion*, 173.

27. Bancroft, "Women Nurses on Wards for Men in Hospitals for the Insane."

28. Charles Bancroft, "Reconciliation of the Disparity between Hospital and Asylum Trained Nurses," *American Journal of Psychiatry* (October 1904): 199–209.

29. McLean Asylum Training School for Nurses, advertising brochure.

30. Bancroft, "Reconciliation of the Disparity between Hospital and Asylum Trained Nurses," 202.

31. Bancroft.

32. These debates are explored in depth in subsequent chapters.

33. The official journal of the APA has had various names, and at the time of Bancroft's writing it was called the *American Journal of Insanity*. To reduce confusion, I refer to it throughout as the *American Journal of Psychiatry*, its current official title.

34. Charles Bancroft, "Report of the Committee on Training Schools for Nurses," *American Journal of Psychiatry* (July 1906): 119–140.

35. The National League for Nursing Education (NLNE) was responsible for the accreditation of formal nurse training courses, but did not have a coherent curriculum statement published until 1917.

36. Bancroft, "Report of the Committee on Training Schools for Nurses," 119.
37. Harry M. Murdock, *A Report to the Rockefeller Foundation on the Psychiatric Nursing Project, July 1, 1942–June 30, 1951*, p1. RAC, RG1.1 Projects, Series 200, Subseries 200A. US Medical Services, box 71, folder 855: American Psychiatric Association, Nursing Reports and Pamphlets, 1945–1951.
38. E. H. Cohoon, "The Responsibility of the American Psychiatric Association in Relation to Psychiatric Nursing," *American Journal of Psychiatry* 79, no. 2 (1922): 211–220.
39. Cohoon, 214.
40. Cohoon, 219.
41. Cohoon.
42. Cohoon, 211.
43. Arthur H. Ruggles, "Psychiatry and the Nurse," *American Journal of Nursing* 26, no. 5 (1926): 357–361.
44. Ruggles, 357.
45. Ruggles.
46. Ruggles, 359.
47. Rubbles, 361.
48. William L. Russell, "The Place of the Nurse in Mental Hygiene," *American Journal of Nursing* 28, no. 9 (1928): 863–870.
49. Russell.
50. A. E. Bennett, "The Value of Psychiatric Training," *American Journal of Nursing* 29, no. 3 (1929): 305.
51. Bennett.
52. Bennett.
53. Bennett.
54. Bennett, 307.

2. "The Gospel of Mental Hygiene"

1. Edith M. Haydon, "Teaching and Supervision of Mental Nursing," *American Journal of Nursing* 28, no. 5 (1928): 499–501.
2. Christine Beebe, "Psychiatry for the Student Nurse," *American Journal of Nursing* 21, no. 7 (1921): 450–454.
3. Beebe.
4. May Kennedy, "Psychiatric Nursing," *American Journal of Nursing* 23, no. 4 (1923): 281.
5. J. H. Ehrenreich, *The Altruistic Imagination: A History of Social Work and Social Policy in the United States* (Ithaca, NY: Cornell University Press, 2014).
6. Gerald N. Grob, *The Mad Among Us: A History of the Care of America's Mentally Ill* (London: Free Press, 1994), 151–164.
7. Grob.
8. Katherine McLean, "Value of Psychiatric Training for Nurses," *American Journal of Nursing* 28, no. 5 (1928): 501–503.
9. Kennedy, "Psychiatric Nursing," 281.
10. Myra Whitney, "The Value of a Brief Course in Psychiatric Nursing," *American Journal of Nursing* 28, no. 5 (1928): 503–505.
11. Louise P. Yale, "Nurses and Suicide Prevention," *American Journal of Nursing* 34, no. 9 (1934): 882–886.
12. Yale, 885.

13. Haydon, "Teaching and Supervision of Mental Nursing," 499.

14. Grob, *Mad Among Us*, 158–159.

15. Patricia D'Antonio, *Nursing with a Message: Public Health Demonstration Projects in New York City* (New Brunswick, NJ: Rutgers University Press, 2017).

16. Dennis Doyle, *Psychiatry and Racial Liberalism in Harlem 1936–1968* (Rochester, NY: University of Rochester Press, 2016), 22. For more in-depth histories of the child guidance movement, see Margo Horn, *Before It's Too Late: The Child Guidance Movement in the United States 1922–1945* (Philadelphia: Temple University Press, 1989); Kathleen Jones, *Taming the Troublesome Child: American Families, Child Guidance and the Limits of Psychiatric Authority* (Cambridge, MA: Harvard University Press, 1999).

17. Horn, *Before It's Too Late*, 58.

18. Effie J. Taylor, "Psychiatry and the Nurse [and Discussion]," *American Journal of Nursing* 26, no. 8 (1926): 634.

19. V. M. Macdonald, "Mental Health of Children: Third Paper: The Growing Mind: Support from Confidence, Stimulus from Success (Continued)," *American Journal of Nursing* 22, no. 3 (1921): 174–176.

20. Macdonald.

21. Jones, *Taming the Troublesome Child*.

22. Grob, *Mad Among Us*, 141–145.

23. Grob.

24. Esther L. Richards, "Is Psychiatric Training Essential to the Equipment of a Graduate Nurse?," *American Journal of Nursing* 22, no. 8 (1922): 629 (emphasis added).

25. Richards.

26. Harriet Bailey, "A Plea for the Inclusion of Mental Nursing in the Training School Curriculum," *American Journal of Nursing* 22, no. 7 (1922): 531–534; Effie J. Taylor, "Course of Study in Practical Psychology and Psychopathology as Given to Student Nurses in the Henry Phipps Psychiatric Clinic, the Johns Hopkins Hospital," *American Journal of Nursing* 22, no. 7 (1922): 534–538.

27. Harriet Bailey, *Nursing Mental Diseases* (New York: Macmillan, 1920).

28. Richards, "Is Psychiatric Training Essential to the Equipment of a Graduate Nurse?"

29. Bailey, *Nursing Mental Diseases*, viii.

30. Bailey, 41.

31. Bailey, "Plea for the Inclusion of Mental Nursing in the Training School Curriculum."

32. Bailey, *Nursing Mental Diseases*, 41.

33. Bailey.

34. Bailey, 42.

35. Bailey, 49.

36. Bailey, 46.

37. Bailey, 47.

38. Elizabeth Lunbeck, *The Psychiatric Persuasion: Knowledge, Gender and Power in Modern America* (Princeton, NJ: Princeton University Press, 1994).

39. Bailey, *Nursing Mental Diseases*, 47.

40. Bailey.

41. Adolf Meyer, "The Philosophy of Occupation Therapy," *Archives of Occupational Therapy* 1 (1922): 1–10.

42. Charles Christiansen, "Adolf Meyer Revisited: Connections between Lifestyles, Resilience and Illness," *Journal of Occupational Science* 14, no. 2 (July 2007): 63–67.

43. Patricia D'Antonio, *Founding Friends: Families, Staff and Patients at the Friends Asylum in Early Nineteenth Century Philadelphia* (Bethlehem, PA: Lehigh Press, 2006).

44. Grob, *Mad Among Us*, 151.

45. Grob, 151.

46. Grob.

47. Ian Robert Dowbiggin, *Keeping America Sane: Psychiatry and Eugenics in the United States and Canada 1880–1940* (Ithaca, NY: Cornell University Press, 2003).

48. Grob, *Mad Among Us*.

49. Bailey, *Nursing Mental Diseases*, 48.

50. Jones, *Taming the Troublesome Child*.

51. Bailey, *Nursing Mental Diseases*, 155.

52. Bailey.

53. Bailey.

54. Grob, *Mad Among Us*.

55. Bailey, Nursing Mental Diseases, 11.

56. Bailey, 11.

57. Grob, *Mad Among Us*, 142.

58. Adolf Meyer, letter to William Healy, cited in Grob, *Mad Among Us*, 143.

59. Grob, *Mad Among Us*, 143.

60. Grob.

61. Bailey, *Nursing Mental Diseases*, 37.

62. Bailey.

63. Grob, *Mad Among Us*.

64. Bailey, *Nursing Mental Diseases*, 40.

65. Bailey, 130.

66. Bailey, 136.

67. Bailey, 146.

68. Bailey, 125.

69. Bailey, 157.

70. Bailey, 19–20.

71. Francis C. Thielbar, "Ward Teaching in a Mental Hospital," *American Journal of Nursing* 41, no. 10 (1941): 710–711.

72. Bailey, "Plea for the Inclusion of Mental Nursing in the Training School Curriculum," 532.

73. Taylor, "Psychiatry and the Nurse [and Discussion]," 631.

74. Taylor.

75. Taylor, 633.

76. Beebe, "Psychiatry for the Student Nurse," 450.

77. Beebe, 452.

78. Kennedy, "Psychiatric Nursing," 279.

79. McLean, "Value of Psychiatric Training for Nurses," 51.

80. Tina Duerksen, "A Psychiatric Viewpoint: For All Nurses," *American Journal of Nursing* 41, no. 11 (1941): 1277–1280.

81. These committees will be explored in chapter 3.

82. May Kennedy, "Psychiatry in Nursing Education," *American Journal of Nursing* 37, no. 10 (1937): 1139–1144.

83. Richards, "Is Psychiatric Training Essential to the Equipment of a Graduate Nurse?," 632.

84. Taylor, "Psychiatry and the Nurse [and Discussion]," 634.

85. Taylor.
86. Taylor.
87. Taylor, 634.
88. Beebe, "Psychiatry for the Student Nurse," 452.
89. Bailey, "Plea for the Inclusion of Mental Nursing in the Training School Curriculum," 534.
90. McLean, "Value of Psychiatric Training for Nurses," 503.
91. Kennedy, "Psychiatric Nursing," 281.
92. Haydon, "Teaching and Supervision of Mental Nursing,"499.
93. Haydon, 499.
94. Whitney, "Value of a Brief Course in Psychiatric Nursing," 505.
95. Thielbar, "Ward Teaching in a Mental Hospital," 710–711.
96. Yale, "Nurses and Suicide Prevention," 886.
97. Yale.
98. Esther Anderson, "Open Road Ahead: In Psychiatric Nursing," *American Journal of Nursing* 41, no. 10 (1941): 1183–1188.
99. Effie J. Taylor, "Twenty-Five Years in Nursing Education: President's Address," *American Journal of Nursing* 35, no. 7 (1935): 653–657.
100. Taylor.
101. Taylor, "Psychiatry and the Nurse [and Discussion]," 634.
102. Bailey, "Plea for the Inclusion of Mental Nursing in the Training School Curriculum," 532.
103. Anderson, "Open Road Ahead," 1184.
104. Anderson, 1183–1188.
105. Anderson.
106. Olga M. Church and Kathleen Coen Buckwalter, "Harriet Bailey—A Psychiatric Nurse Pioneer," *Perspectives in Psychiatric Care* 18, no. 2 (1980): 62–66.

3. "The Nurse of Tomorrow"

1. Esther L. Richards, "Is Psychiatric Training Essential to the Equipment of a Graduate Nurse?" *American Journal of Nursing* 22, no. 8 (1922): 625–632, https://doi.org/10.2307/3406797.
2. *Proceedings of the Twenty-Second Annual Convention of the NLNE* (Baltimore: Williams and Wilkins, 1916).
3. *Proceedings of the Fortieth Annual Convention of the NLNE* (New York: National Headquarters, 1934), 56.
4. Harriet Bailey, "Nursing Schools in Psychiatric Hospitals: A Survey," *American Journal of Nursing* 36, no. 5 (1936): 495–508.
5. Bailey, 495–508.
6. Bailey, 507.
7. Bailey.
8. Bailey, 508.
9. Bailey.
10. Bailey.
11. Bailey.
12. Bailey.
13. Bailey.
14. Bailey.
15. Bailey.

16. Bailey.
17. The question of male psychiatric nurses and the schools that were opening specifically for them will be addressed in chapter 4.
18. Bailey, "Nursing Schools in Psychiatric Hospitals," 811.
19. Bailey.
20. Bailey.
21. Bailey.
22. Isabel M. Stewart, "Advanced Courses in Clinical Subjects," *American Journal of Nursing* 33, no. 6 (1933): 583–589.
23. Anna K. McGibbon and Elizabeth S. Bixler, "An Advanced Course in Psychiatric Nursing," *American Journal of Nursing* 37, no. 2 (1937): 173–180.
24. McGibbon and Bixler, 174.
25. McGibbon and Bixler, 176.
26. McGibbon and Bixler.
27. McGibbon and Bixler, 177.
28. McGibbon and Bixler.
29. McGibbon and Bixler.
30. NLNE, *A Curriculum Guide for Schools of Nursing, Second Revision: Prepared by the Committee on Curriculum of the National League of Nursing Education* (New York: NLNE, 1937).
31. George H. Stevenson, "Psychiatric Nursing Education: Recommended Standards and Curricula for Undergraduate General Nursing Courses in Psychiatric Hospitals, Affiliate and Postgraduate Courses in Psychiatric Nursing," *American Journal of Psychiatry* 96, no. 1 (July 1939): 213–222.
32. Stevenson, 213.
33. Stevenson, 219
34. Stevenson.
35. "Report of the Committee on Curriculum," in *Proceedings of the Forty-Fifth Annual Convention of the NLNE.* (New York: National Headquarters, 1939), 156. Private collection of Sandra Lewenson.
36. "Report of the Committee on Mental Hygiene and Psychiatric Nursing," in *Proceedings of the Forty-Sixth Annual Convention of the NLNE.* (New York: National Headquarters, 1940), 109. Private Collection of Sandra Lewenson.
37. George H. Stevenson, "Ward Personnel in Mental Hospitals," *American Journal of Psychiatry* 91, no. 4 (1935): 791–798.
38. Stevenson, 792.
39. Stevenson, 794–795.
40. Stevenson.
41. Stevenson, 798.
42. Stevenson.
43. Adolf Meyer et al., "Postgraduate Work in Psychiatric Nursing: Five Eminent Psychiatrists Discuss Its Advantages and Values," *American Journal of Nursing* 37, no. 2 (1937): 181–187.
44. William C. Menninger, "Psychiatry in Nursing Education," in *Proceedings of the Forty-Fourth Annual Convention of the NLNE.* (New York: National Headquarters, 1938), 201–209. Private Collection of Sandra Lewenson.
45. Menninger, 208–209.
46. "Report of the Committee on Mental Hygiene and Psychiatric Nursing," in *Proceedings of the Forty-Fourth Annual Convention of the NLNE,* 62–65.

47. "Report of the Committee on Mental Hygiene and Psychiatric Nursing," 64.

48. Charles Fitzpatrick, *Committee on Psychiatric Nursing Interim Semi-Annual Report to the Council*, APA, January 1941, box 70, folder 850, Record Group (RG) 1: Series 200, Rockefeller Foundation (RF), Rockefeller Archive Center, Sleepy Hollow, New York (hereafter referred to as RAC), 2.

49. Fitzpatrick.

50. Fitzpatrick.

51. Fitzpatrick.

52. Alan Gregg, diary excerpt, December 18, 1941, box 70, folder 850, RG 1: Series 200, RF, RAC.

53. Charles Fitzpatrick, letter to Alan Gregg, December 30, 1941, box 70, folder 850, RG 1: Series 200, RF, RAC.

54. Alan Gregg, diary excerpt, June 1942, box 70, folder 851, RG 1: Series 200, RF, RAC.

55. Gregg, diary excerpt, June 1942.

56. Laura Fitzsimmons, letter and report to Alan Gregg, April 12, 1943, 9-10, box 70, folder 851, RG 1: Series 200, RF, RAC.

57. Fitzsimmons to Gregg, April 12, 1943.

58. Fitzsimmons to Gregg, April 12, 1943.

59. Fitzsimmons to Gregg, April 12, 1943.

60. Alan Gregg, diary excerpt, June 18, 1945, box 71, folder 852, RG 1: Series 200, RF, RAC.

61. Laura W. Fitzsimmons, "University Controlled Advanced Clinical Programs in Psychiatric Nursing," *American Journal of Nursing* 44, no. 12 (December 1944): 1166-1169.

62. Fitzsimmons, 1169.

63. Charles Fitzpatrick, letter to Alan Gregg, December 22, 1944, box 71, folder 852, RG 1: Series 200, RF, RAC.

64. Karl Menninger, letter to Robert Morrison, October 8, 1947, box 1, folder 2, RG 1.1 (FA386): Series 219, RF, RAC.

65. Menninger to Morrison, October 8, 1947.

66. Menninger to Morrison, October 8, 1947.

67. Robert Morrison, diary excerpt, January 19, 1949, box 1, folder 4, RG 1.1 (FA386): Series 219, RF, RAC.

68. Robert Morrison, diary excerpt, November 30, 1948, box 1, folder 3, RG 1.1 (FA386): Series 219, RF, RAC.

69. Morrison, diary excerpt, January 19, 1949.

70. Robert Morrison, diary excerpt, September 18, 1951, box 1, folder 5, RG 1.1 Series 219, RF, RAC.

71. Fitzsimmons remained closely involved with nursing organizations activities in relation to psychiatric nursing, which will be explored later in this chapter.

72. Mary Tennant, interoffice memo to Robert Morrison, January 13, 1951, box 71, folder 854, RG 1: Series 200, RF, RAC.

73. Eugenia K. Spalding, "The Bolton Act Provides Federal Funds for Postgraduate Programs," *American Journal of Nursing* 43, no. 9 (1943): 833-834.

74. "Roundtable on Psychiatric Nursing," in *Proceedings of the Forty-Third Annual Convention of the NLNE.* (New York: National Headquarters, 1942), 52. Private Collection of Sandra Lewenson.

75. Hildegard Peplau, "Historical Development of Psychiatric Nursing: A Preliminary Statement of Some Facts and Trends," in *A Collection of Classics in Psychiatric*

Nursing Literature, edited by S. Smoyak and S. Rouslin (Thorofare, NJ: Charles B Slack, 1982), 10–46.

76. NLNE, *Courses in Clinical Nursing for Graduate Nurses: An Advanced Course in Psychiatric Nursing/Prepared by Subcommittee on Psychiatric Nursing of the Special Committee on Postgraduate Clinical Nursing Courses* (New York: NLNE, 1945).
77. NLNE, 1.
78. NLNE, 3.
79. NLNE, 1.
80. NLNE, 1–3.
81. NLNE, 3.
82. NLNE.
83. NLNE, 8.
84. NLNE, 10.
85. NLNE.
86. NLNE.
87. NLNE, 8.
88. NLNE.
89. NLNE, 9
90. NLNE.
91. NLNE.
92. NLNE, 6.

4. "We Called It 'Talking with Patients'"

1. Bosley Crowther, "'Snake Pit,' Study of Mental Ills Based on Mary Jane Ward's Novel, Opens at Rivoli," *New York Times,* November 5, 1948.
2. Editorial, "The Snake Pit," *American Journal of Nursing,* 49, no. 1 (1949): 2.
3. Vern L. Bullough, and Lilli Sentz, eds., *American Nursing: A Biographical Dictionary,* vol. 3. (New York: Springer, 2004), 97.
4. Mary M. Schmitt, "Some Weaknesses and Strengths of Present-Day Psychiatric Nursing Programs," *American Journal of Nursing* 49, no. 8 (1949): 531–534.
5. Schmitt.
6. Esther Garrison, "Psychiatric Nursing Education Program Developments," *Psychiatric Services* 4, no. 10 (December 1953): 14–15.
7. Garrison.
8. The full conference proceedings have not been published but are summarized in Hildegard Peplau, "Historical Development of Psychiatric Nursing: A Preliminary Statement of Some Facts and Trends," in *A Collection of Classics in Psychiatric Nursing Literature,* edited by S. Smoyak and S. Rousin (Thorofare, NJ: Charles B. Slack, 1982), 10–46.
9. Peplau.
10. Claire Mintzer Fagin, *A Study of Desirable Functions and Qualifications for Psychiatric Nurses* (New York: NLNE; National Organization of Public Health Nursing, 1953).
11. Mintzer Fagin, 9.
12. Mintzer Fagin, 10.
13. Mintzer Fagin, 28.
14. Mintzer Fagin, 30.
15. Mintzer Fagin, 29.
16. Mintzer Fagin, 33.

17. Mintzer Fagin, 34.
18. Helena Willis Render, *Nurse-Patient Relationships in Psychiatry* (New York: McGraw-Hill, 1947).
19. Willis Render, 4.
20. Willis Render, 9–10
21. Willis Render, 11.
22. Willis Render, 19.
23. Suzanne Lego, "The One-to-One Nurse Patient Relationship," in *Psychiatric Nursing 1946 to 1974: A Report on the State of the Art* (New York: American Journal of Nursing, 1975), 1–14.
24. Lego, 2
25. Barbara J. Callaway, *Hildegard Peplau: Psychiatric Nurse of the Century* (New York: Springer, 2002).
26. Peplau, "Historical Development of Psychiatric Nursing," 23.
27. Hildegard Peplau, "Oral History, Psychiatric Nursing Career," ed. Patricia D'Antonio, 1985, box 1, folder 2, HEP Papers.
28. Peplau.
29. Callaway, *Hildegard Peplau*, 61–62.
30. Callaway, 76–80
31. Hildegard E. Peplau Papers, Schlesinger Library Collection, Radcliffe Institute for the Study of American Women, Harvard University, Cambridge, Massachusetts (hereafter referred to as HEP Papers SLC), carton 9, files 277, 278v, 283v, 285v, 286, 287v.
32. Callaway, *Hildegard Peplau*, 61–62.
33. William Menninger, *Psychiatry in a Troubled World* (New York: Macmillan, 1948).
34. U.S. Army Medical Department, *Neuropsychiatry in World War II* (Washington, DC: 1966–1973); Menninger, *Psychiatry in a Troubled World*; Callaway, *Hildegard Peplau*; Gerald N. Grob, *From Asylum to Community: Mental Health Policy in Modern America* (Princeton, NJ: Princeton University Press, 1991).
35. Hildegard Peplau, letter to Bertha Peplau, July 1, 1944, carton 3, file 60-64, HEP Papers SLC.
36. Peplau to Peplau, July 1, 1944.
37. Peplau, "Oral History, Psychiatric Nursing Career."
38. Peplau.
39. Peplau.
40. Interview with Claire Fagin by Susan Reverby, August 1982, box 30, Claire M. Fagin Papers, MC 95, Barbara Bates Center for the Study of the History of Nursing, School of Nursing, University of Pennsylvania, p. 100.
41. Callaway, *Hildegard Peplau*, 157.
42. Peplau, "Oral History, Psychiatric Nursing Career."
43. Hildegard Peplau, *Interpersonal Relations in Nursing: A Conceptual Frame of Reference for Psychodynamic Nursing* (New York: G. P. Putnam's Sons, 1952).
44. Interview with Claire Fagin, 105.
45. Callaway, *Hildegard Peplau*, 224–225.
46. Peplau, "Oral History, Psychiatric Nursing Career."
47. Peplau.
48. Hildegard Peplau, "Interpersonal Techniques: The Crux of Psychiatric Nursing," *American Journal of Nursing* 62, no. 6 (1962): 50–54; Hildegard Peplau, "Present Day Trends in Psychiatric Nursing," *Neuropsychiatry* 3 (1963): 190–204; Hildegard Peplau, "Talking with Patients," *American Journal of Nursing* 60, no. 7 (1960): 964–966;

Hildegard Peplau, "Interpersonal Relations and the Process of Adaptation," *Nursing Science* 1, no. 4 (1960): 272–279.

49. Peplau, "Present Day Trends."
50. Gerald N. Grob, *The Mad Among Us: A History of the Care of America's Mentally Ill* (London: Free Press, 1994).
51. Peplau, "Present Day Trends."
52. Peplau.
53. Peplau.
54. Peplau, *Interpersonal Relations in Nursing*.
55. Dorothy Mereness, "Oral History," March 26, 1985, ed. Patricia D'Antonio, box 1, folder 1, Dorothy A. Mereness Papers, MC 55, Barbara Bates Center for the Study of the History of Nursing, School of Nursing, University of Pennsylvania, Philadelphia (hereafter cited as DAM Papers BBC).
56. Mereness, "Oral History."
57. Mereness, "Oral History."
58. Mereness, "Oral History."
59. Mereness, "Oral History."
60. Dorothy Mereness, "Preparation of the Nurse for the Psychiatric Team," *American Journal of Nursing* 51, no. 5 (1951): 320–322.
61. Mereness, 320.
62. Mereness, "Oral History."
63. Mereness, "Preparation of the Nurse," 321.
64. Mereness, "Oral History."
65. Mereness, "Oral History."
66. Mereness, "Oral History."
67. Mereness, "Oral History."
68. Mereness, "Oral History."
69. Mereness, "Oral History."
70. Mereness, "Oral History."
71. Dorothy Mereness, "Family Therapy: An Evolving Role for the Psychiatric Nurse," speech given at the Yale University School of Nursing Psychiatric Conference, April 20, 1967, box 1, folder 9, DAM Papers BBC.
72. Dorothy Mereness, "Psychotherapeutic Nursing: The Meaning, Need and Role of Nursing in the Practice of Therapeutic Nursing," speech given at the Veterans Administration (VA) Hospital, Topeka, Kansas, May 25, 1967, box 1, folder 9, DAM Papers BBC.
73. Dorothy Mereness, "Factors Influencing the Psychiatric Nurse's Role and Function," Unpublished Paper, c. 1958, box 1, folder 7, DAM Papers BBC.
74. Mereness. Milieu therapy refers to the idea that the living environment of the patient should be itself deliberately therapeutic, which had loosely informed psychiatry for some time. It became a more formal theory in American psychiatry with the development of "therapeutic communities" from the 1950s. Grob, *The Mad Among Us*, 226–228.
75. Mereness, "Oral History."
76. Dorothy Mereness, "The Role of the Psychiatric Nurse in Therapy," speech given at Montrose VA Hospital, New York, June 1963, box 1, folder 8, DAM Papers BBC.
77. Mereness.
78. Gwen E. Tudor, "A Sociopsychiatric Nursing Approach to Intervention in a Problem of Mutual Withdrawal on a Mental Hospital Ward," *Psychiatry: Interpersonal and Biological Processes* 15, no. 2 (1952): 193–217.

79. Schwartz himself was interested in the role of the nurse in therapeutic relations and went on to publish the book *The Nurse and the Mental Patient: A Study in Interpersonal Relations* (New York: Russell Sage Foundation, 1956).

80. Tudor, "Sociopsychiatric Nursing Approach to Intervention in a Problem of Mutual Withdrawal on a Mental Hospital Ward," 193.

81. Tudor.

82. Tudor, 194.

83. Tudor, 216.

84. Tudor, 217.

85. Tudor.

86. Peplau, "Historical Development of Psychiatric Nursing," 38.

87. Group for the Advancement of Psychiatry (GAP), *Therapeutic Use of Self: A Concept for Teaching Patient Care* (New York: GAP, 1955).

88. Helen Nakagawa, "Group Theory in Nursing Practice," in *Psychiatric Nursing 1946 to 1974: A Report on the State of the Art*, ed. Florence L. Huey (New York: American Journal of Nursing, 1976), 15–21.

89. Ildaura Murillo-Rohde, biographical note, Box 1, Ildaura Murillo-Rohde Papers, MC 172, Barbara Bates Center for the Study of the History of Nursing, School of Nursing, University of Pennsylvania (hereafter IMR Papers BBC).

90. Murillo-Rohde.

91. Claire M. Fagin, interview with author, September 15, 2017, New York City.

92. Hildegard Peplau, handwritten note, VA Meeting, October 1954, Carton 20,unnumbered file. HEP Papers SLC.

93. June Mellow, "Research in Nursing Therapy," in *The Improvement of Nursing through Research* (Washington, DC: Catholic University of America Press, 1958), 110–112.

94. Alice Robinson et al., "Research in Psychiatric Nursing 1: The Role of the Nurse Therapist in a Large Public Mental Hospital," *American Journal of Nursing* 55, no. 4 (1955): 441–443; June Mellow et al., "Research in Psychiatric Nursing 2: Nursing Therapy with Individual Patients," *American Journal of Nursing* 55, no. 5 (1955): 572–575; Mellow, "Research in Nursing Therapy."

95. Mellow, "Research in Nursing Therapy."

96. Mellow.

97. Robinson et al., "Research in Psychiatric Nursing 1."

98. Hildegard Peplau, Panel Discussion Transcript, April 1968, Carton 25, Files 903 and 904, HEP Papers SLC.

99. Elizabeth Pittman, *Luther Christman: A Maverick Nurse—a Nursing Legend* (Bloomington, IN: Trafford, 2005).

100. Mereness, "Role of the Psychiatric Nurse in Therapy."

101. Dorothy Mereness, "The Nurse's Developing Role in Community Psychiatry," speech given at Little Rock VA Hospital, March 1967, box 1, folder 9, DAM Papers BBC.

102. Mereness, "Psychotherapeutic Nursing."

103. Mereness.

104. Mereness, "Family Therapy."

105. Mereness, "Psychotherapeutic Nursing."

106. Shirley A. Smoyak, "Family Therapy," in Huey, *Psychiatric Nursing 1946 to 1974*, 36–49.

107. Claire M. Fagin. "Why Not Involve Parents When Children Are Hospitalized?" *American Journal of Nursing* 62, no. 6 (1962): 78–79.

108. Murillo-Rohde, biographical note.

109. Murillo-Rohde.
110. Ildaura Murillo-Rohde, "The Nurse as Family Therapist," *Nursing Outlook* 16 (May 1968): 49–52; Barbara Brush and Antonia Villaruel, "Heeding the Past, Leading the Future," *Hispanic Health Care International* 12, no. 4 (2014): 159–160. Murillo-Rohde's work on the intersection of race, culture, and mental health will be explored in greater depth in chapter 5.
111. This was a much-discussed issue in nursing and psychiatry journals from the late 1940s onward. See, for example, Robert H. Felix, "Mental Hygiene and Public Health," *American Journal of Orthopsychiatry* 18 (1948): 679–684; Winifred M. Geisel, "The Psychiatric Nurse in the Community," *American Journal of Nursing* 49, no. 1 (1949): 23–24; Frances Henderson, "The Nurse in a Mental Health Clinic," *Public Health Nursing* 41 (1949): 42–45; James Plant, "The Public Health Nurse as a Medium for Mental Health," *Public Health Nursing* 39 (1947): 3–6; Pearl Shalit, "The Psychiatric Nurse in a Community Mental Health Program," *American Journal of Nursing* 48, no. 11 (1948): 377–380.
112. Hildegard Peplau, "The Work of Psychiatric Nurses," speech (location unknown), November 1966, box 3, folder 53, HEP Papers BBC.
113. Hildegard Peplau, "Public Health Nursing: A Community Resource for Promoting Mental Health," speech given at the Sommerset Visiting Nurses Association, New Jersey, 1959, box 2 folder 2, HEP Papers BBC.
114. Peplau.
115. Robert H. Felix, "Mental Disorders as a Public Health Problem," *American Journal of Psychiatry* 106, no. 6 (1949): 401–406.
116. Peplau, "Public Health Nursing."
117. Hildegard Peplau, "Therapeutic Functions," speech given at Regional Conference of the NLNE, 1956, box 2, folder 26, HEP Papers BBC.
118. Hildegard Peplau, "Interpersonal Relations in Nursing," speech given to TriState Hospital Associations Annual Nursing Service Institute, Delaware State Hospital, New Castle, March 18, 1964, box 2, folder 2, HEP Papers BBC.
119. Hildegard Peplau, "Psychiatric Aspects of Nursing Practice," speech given at the Eighth Annual Convention of the New Jersey League for Nursing, October 5, 1960, box 2, folder 34, HEP Papers BBC.
120. Peplau, "Public Health Nursing."
121. Hildegard Peplau, "The Nurse in the Community Mental Health Program," *Nursing Outlook* 13, no. 11 (1965): 68–70.
122. Menninger, *Psychiatry in a Troubled World.*
123. Fromm, *Escape from Freedom.*
124. Peplau, "Oral History, Psychiatric Nursing Career."
125. Peplau, "Talking with Patients."
126. Grayce Sills, "Research in the Field of Psychiatric Nursing," *Nursing Research* 26, no. 3 (1977): 201–207.

5. "The Number One Social Problem"

1. Hildegard Peplau, "Current Concepts of Psychiatric Nursing," speech given to the ANA Convention, Atlantic City, New Jersey, June 11, 1958, box 2, folder 30, HEP Papers BBC.
2. Gerald N. Grob, *From Asylum to Community: Mental Health Policy in Modern America* (Princeton, NJ: Princeton University Press, 1991); Nathan G. Hale, *Freud and the*

Americans: The Beginnings of Psychoanalysis in the United States 1876–1917 (Oxford: Oxford University Press, 1971).

3. Hildegard Peplau, "Mental Health and the Public Pulse," speech given at New York University, December 7, 1972, box 3, folder 65, HEP Papers BBC.

4. Peplau. See also Albert Deutsch, *The Story of GAP* (New York: GAP, 1959).

5. Erich Fromm, *Escape from Freedom* (New York: Holt, Rinehart, and Winston, 1941).

6. William Menninger, *Psychiatry in a Troubled World* (New York: Macmillan, 1948).

7. Rollo May, *The Meaning of Anxiety* (New York: Ronald Press, 1950); Alexander Leighton, John Clausen, and Robert Wilson, eds., *Explorations in Social Psychiatry* (London: Tavistock, 1957).

8. Kyle. A. Cuordileone, "Politics in an Age of Anxiety: Cold War Political Culture and the Crisis in American Masculinity, 1949–1960," *Journal of American History* 87, no. 2 (2000): 515–545.

9. Fromm, *Escape from Freedom*; Abram Kardiner, *The Traumatic Neuroses of War* (Washington, DC: National Academies, 1941); John Dollard et al., *Frustration and Aggression* (New Haven, CT: Yale University Press, 1939).

10. Arthur Schlesinger Jr., *The Vital Center: The Politics of Freedom* (Boston: Houghton Mifflin, 1949)

11. Rollo May, *The Meaning of Anxiety*, rev. ed. (New York: Norton, 1977).

12. May, 10–11.

13. Hildegard Peplau, "The Work of Psychiatric Nurses," speech (location unknown), November 1966, box 3 folder 53, HEP Papers BBC.

14. Hildegard Peplau, "Public Health Nursing: A Community Resource for Promoting Mental Health," speech given at Somerset Visiting Nurses Association, New Jersey, 1959, box 2, folder 2, HEP Papers BBC.

15. Peplau, "Current Concepts of Psychiatric Nursing."

16. Hildegard Peplau, "Present Day Trends in Psychiatric Nursing," *Neuropsychiatry* 3 (1963): 190–204.

17. Hildegard Peplau, "Leadership Responsibility in Toleration of Stress," speech given at Teachers College, Columbia University, June 7, 1963, box 2, folder 37, HEP Papers BBC.

18. Dorothy Mereness, "The Nurse as an Individual in a Changing World," speech delivered at an afternoon NLNE meeting in New York City, c. 1958, box 1, folder 7, DAM Papers BBC.

19. Mereness.

20. Dorothy Mereness, "Factors Influencing the Psychiatric Nurse's Role and Function," c. 1958, unpublished paper, box 1, folder 7, DAM Papers BBC.

21. Mereness.

22. Mereness.

23. Mereness.

24. Hildegard Peplau, "Oral History, Psychiatric Nursing Career," ed. Patricia D'Antonio, 1985, box 1, folder 2, HEP Papers BBC.

25. Menninger, *Psychiatry in a Troubled World*; Cuordileone, "Politics in an Age of Anxiety."

26. Hildegard Peplau, "A Bold New Approach," May 1965, unpublished manuscript, box 3, folder 52, HEP Papers BBC.

27. Hildegard Peplau, "Trends in Psychiatric-Mental Health Nursing," speech given at ANA Clinical Sessions, 1962, box 2, folder 36, HEP Papers BBC.

28. Dennis Doyle, *Psychiatry and Racial Liberalism in Harlem, 1936–1968* (Rochester, NY: University of Rochester Press, 2016); Michael Staub, *The Mismeasure of Minds: Debating Race and Intelligence between Brown and the Bell Curve* (Chapel Hill: University of North Carolina Press, 2018).

29. Jay Garcia, *Psychology Comes to Harlem: Rethinking the Race Question in Twentieth-Century America* (Baltimore: Johns Hopkins University Press, 2012); Gabriel N. Mendes, *Under the Strain of Color: Harlem's Lafargue Clinic and the Promise of an Antiracist Psychiatry* (Ithaca, NY: Cornell University Press, 2015); Doyle, *Psychiatry and Racial Liberalism in Harlem, 1936–1968.*

30. Darlene Clark Hine, *Black Women in White: Racial Conflict and Cooperation in the Nursing Profession 1890–1950* (Bloomington: University of Indiana Press, 1989); Charissa Threat, *Nursing Civil Rights: Gender and Race in the Army Nurse Corps* (Chicago: University of Illinois Press, 2015).

31. Alma Jones, letter to Mabel Staupers, box 2, folder 2, National Association of Colored Graduate Nurses (NACGN) records, Schomburg Center for Research in Black Culture, New York Public Library (hereafter NACGN Records SC).

32. Mabel Staupers, letter to Alma Jones, June 9, 1942, box 2, folder 2, NACGN Records SC.

33. Mabel Staupers, letter to William T. Andrews, June 27, 1942, box 2, folder 2, NACGN Records SC. Blanks in this instance refers to blank employment application forms for state positions.

34. Darlene Clark Hine and Katherine Thompson, *Facts on File Encyclopedia of Black Women in America* (New York: Facts on File, 1997).

35. Ruth Logan Roberts, letter to Thomas E. Dewey, October 22, 1942, box 2, folder 2, NACGN Records SC.

36. John Bennett, letter to Ruth Logan Roberts, October 26, 1942, box 2, folder 2, NACGN Records SC.

37. Ildaura Murillo-Rohde, "Ethnic Minorities in Psychiatric Nursing: Patients and Personnel," November 19, 1982, box 5, IMR Papers BBC. Murillo-Rohde's paper does not mention Native American nurses, reflecting their general omission from both nursing practice and nursing history.

38. Murillo-Rohde.

39. Murillo-Rohde.

40. Murillo-Rohde.

41. Murillo-Rohde.

42. Murillo-Rohde.

43. Jeanne Spurlock, *Black Psychiatrists and American Psychiatry* (Washington, DC: APA, 1999).

44. Spurlock.

45. Prince Barker, "Psychiatry at the Tuskegee VA Hospital in Retrospect," *Journal of the National Medical Association* 54, no. 2 (1962): 152–153.

46. Hine, *Black Women in White.*

47. Genevieve Bixler and Leo Simmons, *The Regional Project in Graduate Education and Research in Nursing* (Atlanta, GA: Southern Regional Education Board [SREB], 1960).

48. SREB, *Mental Health Training and Research in the Southern States* (Atlanta, GA: SREB, 1954).

49. SREB.

50. SREB.

51. SREB.

52. SREB.

53. SREB, *Today and Tomorrow: Summary Report of a Panel on Organization and Conduct on State Mental Health Programs* (Atlanta, GA: SREB, 1956); SREB, *Mental Health Training and Research in the Southern States.*

54. Esther Garrison, letter to Hildegard Peplau, May 1954, carton 20, file 678, HEP Papers SLC.

55. Various notecards, SREB, Daytona Beach, Florida, 1954, carton, 20, file 680, HEP Papers SLC.

56. "Summary of Resolutions," Nursing Group, Southern Regional Conference on Mental Health Training and Research, July 22, 1954, carton 20, file 680, HEP Papers SLC.

57. Virginia Crenshaw to Hildegard Peplau, September 7, 1954, carton 20, file 680, HEP Papers SLC.

58. Hildegard Peplau, unsigned note, carton 20, file 683, HEP Papers SLC.

59. SREB, *Nursing Personnel for Mental Health Programs: Report of a Conference Sponsored by the Southern Regional Education Board* (Atlanta, GA: SREB, 1957).

60. Hildegard Peplau, letter to SREB, June 1957, carton 21, file 724, HEP Papers SLC.

61. Peplau to SREB.

62. Series 20.4, folder 1.13, University of Alabama at Birmingham (UAB) Archives, Birmingham, Alabama (hereafter UAB Archives).

63. *Report of the Trustees of the Alabama State Hospitals (for Mental and Nervous Diseases) to the Governor with Annual Report of the Superintendent for the Year Ending September 30, 1956* (Tuscaloosa, AL: Alabama State Hospitals, 1956).

64. Florence Hixson, *Annual Report: School of Nursing* (Tuscaloosa, AL: University of Alabama, 1958–1959), Series 20.1, folder 1.9, UAB Archives; Seminar on Clinical Aspects of Graduate Programs in Nursing, carton 21, File 738, HEP Papers SLC.

65. Florence Hixson, *Annual Report: School of Nursing* (Tuscaloosa, AL: University of Alabama, 1957–1958), Series 20.1, folder 1.8, UAB Archives, p. 4.

66. Florence Hixson, *Annual Report: School of Nursing* (Tuscaloosa, AL: University of Alabama, 1958–1959), Series 20.1, folder 1.9, UAB Archives.

67. Florence Hixson, *Annual Report: School of Nursing* (Tuscaloosa, AL: University of Alabama, 1965–1966), Series 20.1, folder 1.16, UAB Archives.

68. Florence Hixson, *Annual Report: School of Nursing* (Tuscaloosa, AL: University of Alabama, 1962–1963), Series 20.1, folder 1.13, UAB Archives.

69. Arthur Ree Campbell, "Oral History," School of Nursing History Project, Series M2000-22, folder 1.28, UAB Archives.

70. These memos are contained in Docket No. MCR44, U.S. District Court, Montgomery, Alabama, Civil Case Files, 74-C-0813, box 149, National Archives and Records Administration, Atlanta (hereafter cited as MCR44).

71. Prince Barker, memo to James Tarwater, July 19, 1965, Document GC9Y9, MCR44.

72. Elsie Smith, memo to James Tarwater, July 19, 1965, Document GC9Y9, MCR44.

73. Mrs. Snow, memo to James Tarwater, July 12, 1965, Document GC9Z6, MCR44.

74. District Judge Johnson, Decision, *Marable v. Alabama Mental Health Board v. Finch & United States v. State of Alabama*, Civil Action Nos. 2615-N, 2610-N [297 F. Supp. 293], February 11, 1969, https://law.justia.com/cases/federal/district-courts/FSupp /297/291/2147439/. See also Kylie M. Smith, "The Crippling Preoccupation with Race: Psychiatry and Civil Rights in Alabama," *Journal of Southern History*, forthcoming.

75. Paul Davis, "*Wyatt v. Stickney*: Did We Get It Right This Time?," *Law & Psychology Review* 35 (2011): 143–165; Clifton Slaten, "The 1995 Wyatt Litigation: Beginnings, Trial Strategies, and Results," *Law & Psychology Review* 35 (2011): 179–191; Jack Drake, "Drafting the Case: The Parallel Legacies of *Wyatt v. Stickney* and *Lynch v. Baxley*," *Law & Psychology Review* 35 (2011): 167–177.

76. Slaten, "1995 Wyatt Litigation"; Drake, "Drafting the Case."

77. Davis, "*Wyatt v. Stickney*."

78. Workshop Advisory Group for the Alabama Division of Mental Health, *A Program of Transitional Services for the Mentally Ill: A Collaborative Effort between the Alabama Dept of Mental Health and the Dept of Pensions and Security of the State of Alabama (Evaluation—Pre-Release—Transitional Services)* (Montgomery, AL: Department of Pensions and Security and the Alabama Mental Health Board, June 20, 1972), carton 27, file 1008, HEP Papers SLC.

79. Stonewall Stickney, *Philosophy and Goals of the Department* (Montgomery, AL: State Department of Mental Health, 1970).

80. Workshop Advisory Group for Alabama Division of Mental Health, *Program of Transitional Services for the Mentally Ill*.

Conclusion

1. These changes and their complex intersections have been explored in more detail by a number of scholars. See, for example, Anne E. Parsons, *From Asylum to Prison: Deinstitutionalization and the Rise of Mass Incarceration after 1945* (Chapel Hill: University of North Carolina Press, 2018); Bernard E. Harcourt, "From the Asylum to the Prison: Rethinking the Incarceration Revolution," *Texas Law Review* 84 (June 2006): 1751–1786; Olga Maranjian Church, "From Custody to Community in Psychiatric Nursing," *Nursing Research* 36, no. 1 (1987): 48–55; Gerald N. Grob, *From Asylum to Community: Mental Health Policy in Modern America* (Princeton, NJ: Princeton University Press, 1991); Nancy Tomes, "The Patient as a Policy Factor: A Historical Case Study of the Consumer/Survivor Movement in Mental Health," *Health Affairs* 25, no. 3 (2006): 720–729; Andrew Scull, *Decarceration: Community Treatment and the Deviant: A Radical View*, 2nd ed. (New Brunswick, NJ: Rutgers University Press, 1984); Stephen J. Taylor, *Acts of Conscience: World War II, Mental Institutions, and Religious Objectors* (Syracuse, NY: Syracuse University Press, 2009).

2. A very small sample of this work includes Michael Rice, "Psychiatric Mental Health Evidence-Based Practice," *Journal of the American Psychiatric Nurses Association* 14, no. 2 (2008): 107–111; J. Cahill, G. Paley, and G. Hardy, "What Do Patients Find Helpful in Psychotherapy? Implications for the Therapeutic Relationship in Mental Health Nursing," *Journal of Psychiatric and Mental Health Nursing* 20, no. 9 (2013): 782–791; Janet G. Baradell and Barbara R. Bordeaux, "Outcomes and Satisfaction of Patients of Psychiatric Clinical Nurse Specialists," *Journal of the American Psychiatric Nurses Association* 7, no. 3 (2001): 67–75; Susan McCabe, "Bringing Psychiatric Nursing into the Twenty-First Century," *Archives of Psychiatric Nursing* 14, no. 3 (2000): 109–116.

3. Alisa Roth, *Insane: America's Criminal Treatment of the Mentally Ill* (New York: Basic Books Inc, 2018); Dinah Miller and Annette Hanson, *Committed: The Battle over Involuntary Psychiatric Care* (Baltimore: Johns Hopkins University Press, 2016); J. M. Metzl and K. T. MacLeish, "Mental Illness, Mass Shootings, and the Politics of American Firearms," *American Journal of Public Health* 105, no. 2 (2015): 240–249;

J. M. Metzl and K. T. MacLeish, "Triggering the Debate: Faulty Associations between Violence and Mental Illness Underlie US Gun Control Efforts," *Risk and Regulation* 25 (2013): 8–10.

4. Hildegard Peplau, "Mental Health and the Public Pulse," speech given at New York University, December 7, 1972, box 3, folder 65, HEP Papers BBC. All subsequent quotations are from this speech, which is unpaginated.

Epilogue

1. Mary Starke Harper Papers, MC 150, Barbara Bates Center for the Study of the History of Nursing, School of Nursing, University of Pennsylvania, Philadelphia (hereafter MSH Papers BBC).
2. Dennis McLellan, "Mary S. Harper, 86; Expert on Mental Health, Aging Lamented Role in Tuskegee Syphilis Study," *Los Angeles Times*, August 5, 2006; Matt Schudel, "Mary Harper; Leader in Minority Health," *Washington Post*, August 5, 2006; Priscilla Ebersole, "Mary Harper: Nurse/Politician Extraordinaire," *Geriatric Nursing* 18, no. 4 (1997): 175–177; George Niederehe, "Mary Starke Harper (1919–2006)," *American Psychologist* 62, no. 9 (2007): 1071.
3. Mary Starke Harper, *Human experimentation and the Tuskegee Syphilis Story*, unpublished paper, April 2005. In this paper, Harper also references a speech she gave at Yale University School of Medicine on February 18, 2002, where she also makes this claim; box 10, MSH papers, BBC.
4. Mary Starke Harper, "The Young Veteran Vis-à-vis the Veterans of The Three Previous Crises And/Or Wars" speech presented at 15th Annual Conference VA Cooperative Studies in Psychiatry, Shamrock Hilton Hotel Houston Texas April 2–4 1970. File: "Veterans Administration Co-Operative Research," box 8, MSH Papers BBC.
5. "Veterans Administration Co-Operative Research."
6. Folder: "NIMH Workshop for Minority Fellowship Program Interns," box 9, MSH Papers BBC.
7. Mary Starke Harper, "An Overview of the Centre for the Study of Minority Group Mental Health Programs, National Institute of Mental Health," unpublished report, box 9, MSH Papers BBC.
8. Shirley Smoyak, personal communication, February 2016.
9. Mary Starke Harper, "Emotional, Social and Behavioral Problems of the Elderly and Aging," paper presented at the Psychosocial Well-Being of the Aging Mississippian Workshop, Sanatorium, Mississippi, Tuesday, May 6, 1986, box 1, MSH Papers BBC.
10. Starke Harper.
11. Starke Harper.
12. Mary Starke Harper, "Ethical Issues on Mental Health Research from a Minority Perspective," paper presented at the National Minority Conference on Human Experimentation, Reston, Virginia, January 6–8, 1976, box 1, MSH Papers BBC.
13. Mary Starke Harper, "Racism and Mental Health," policy paper, box 1, MSH Papers BBC.
14. Draft of chapter "Psychosocial Care for Racial and Ethnic Minority Elderly," box 1, MSH Papers BBC.
15. Mary Starke Harper, "The Black Elderly," paper presented at the Fourth Annual Black Experience Workshop, University of North Carolina, Chapel Hill, Friday, March 25, 1983, box 1, MSH Papers BBC.
16. Starke Harper, "Racism and Mental Health."

17. Mildred S. Cannon and Ben Z. Locke, "Being Black Is Detrimental to One's Mental Health: Myth or Reality?," paper presented at the W.E.B. Dubois Conference on the Health of Black Populations, December 14, 1976, Atlanta University, Atlanta, Georgia, box 9, MSH Papers BBC. This paper was eventually published as Mildred S. Cannon and Ben Z. Locke, "Being Black Is Detrimental to One's Mental Health: Myth or Reality?," *Phylon* 38, no. 4 (1977): 408–428.

18. Cannon and Locke, 22.

Index

Page numbers in *italics* represent photographs.

Dewey, Thomas E., 115
Diagnostic and Statistical Manual: Mental Disorders (DSM-I), 8–9
Dibble, Eugene, 118
dictatorships and anxiety, 111
Dillard University (Louisiana), 117–118, 124
Dohlstrom, Arthur, 125, 126–127
Doyle, Dennis, 33
DSM-I. See *Diagnostic and Statistical Manual: Mental Disorders*
Duerksen, Tina, 45
Duke University (North Carolina), 121
Dutter, Elizabeth, 126–127

economic stability/instability, 48, 49, 53, 75. *See also* Great Depression
ECT. *See* electroconvulsive therapy
education. *See* nursing education
electroconvulsive therapy (ECT), 100
electroshock therapy (EST), 100. *See also* shock therapy
Elmhurst General Hospital (New York), 104
Emory University (Georgia), 121, 124
environmental factors. *See* mental health/illness
Escape from Freedom (Erich Fromm), 110
Essentials of Psychiatric Nursing (Mereness), 92
EST. *See* electroshock therapy
eugenics, 38–39, 50, 132

Faber, Marian, 54
Fagin, Claire Mintzer, 81, 82, 83–84, 89, 97, 99, 100, 103–104, 122
family, focus on, 31–34, 36–37, 75, 95, 102–106, 113
family therapy, 96–97, 103
fascism, nature of, 6
Felix, Robert, 4, 105, 120
Ferrier, Marie, 22
fever treatment, 76
Fisk University, 120
Fitzpatrick, Charles, 65–72
Fitzsimmons, Laura Wood, 66–69, 71, 73, 77, 80, 88, 120, 121
Florida A&M University: School of Nursing, 117, 124

Fordism technique, 37
Fort, Ada, 124
Foth, Thomas, 13
Foucault, Michel, 12
Fowles, Carolyn, 88
Freud, Anna, 104
Freud, Sigmund, 6–7, 34, 37, 40, 92, 93, 113
Friends Asylum (Pennsylvania), 15
Fromm, Erich, 9, 86, 87, 110
Fromm-Reichmann, Frida, 9, 87, 88, 90, 92
Fuller, Daniel, 54

GAP. *See* Group for the Advancement of Psychiatry
Garrison, Esther, 80–81, 84, 88, 120–121, 123
Gastaldo, Denise, 13
Gault, Alma, 124
gender: assumptions of care, 8, 14–15, 58; changing role of women, 112–113 (*see also* women's rights); conflicts, 5–6; in early psychiatric nursing, 17–20, 27, 57–58; in interpersonal relations, 102; multiple subjectivities for women, 11–13; stereotypes, 7, 9, 18, 102
GI Bill, 77, 80, 88
Gipe, Florence, 124
Goddard, Henry, 39
Goffman, Erving, 133
Government Hospital for the Insane (Washington, D.C.), 17
Grady Hospital School of Nursing (Atlanta), 117
Great Depression, 32, 48, 54
Gregg, Alan, 65–66, 67, 68, 69
Greystone Park Psychiatric Hospital (New Jersey), 90
Grob, Gerald, 10, 38, 40
Group for the Advancement of Psychiatry (GAP), 69, 98, 110
group therapy, 96–97, 99

Hall, Bernard H., 71, *71*
Halliwell, Martin, 6, 8, 146n4
haloperidol, 138
Harder, Daisy, 54
Harlem Hospital (New York), 114
Harper, Mary Starke, 121, 135–140, *137*

About the Author

Kylie M. Smith is an assistant professor and the Andrew W. Mellon Faculty Fellow in the Nell Hodgson Woodruff School of Nursing at Emory University in Atlanta. Originally from Australia, Dr. Smith holds a PhD in the history of psychiatry and is the coeditor of two volumes on critical theory and nursing history. At Emory she teaches history, ethics, and social justice in the School of Nursing and in the History Department.

Available titles in the Critical Issues in Health and Medicine series:

Printed in the United States
By Bookmasters